Nanomaterial Safety in the Workplace

Pilot Project for Assessing the
Impact of the NIOSH Nanotechnology
Research Center

Eric Landree, Hirokazu Miyake, Victoria A. Greenfield

Prepared for the National Institute for Occupational Safety and Health

For more information on this publication, visit www.rand.org/t/RR1108

Library of Congress Cataloging-in-Publication Data is available for this publication.
ISBN: 978-0-8330-9232-8

Published by the RAND Corporation, Santa Monica, Calif.

© Copyright 2015 RAND Corporation

RAND® is a registered trademark.

Cover image via Ronny Marx/Fotolia

Support RAND

Make a tax-deductible charitable contribution at
www.rand.org/giving/contribute

www.rand.org

Preface

Over the past ten years, the National Institute for Occupational Safety and Health (NIOSH) Nanotechnology Research Center (NTRC), a virtual center set up within the institute, has directed, funded, or helped influence the efforts of more than 90 researchers, including both NIOSH and extramural researchers. These efforts have contributed to hundreds of scientific articles and facilitated engagement with industry and other stakeholders to promote the safety and health of workers who might come in contact with nanoscale materials; however, the extent to which those efforts have contributed to improvements in worker safety and health through changes in workplace practices and the reduction of workplace-related injuries, illnesses, or fatalities has not yet been established.

In August 2014, the RAND Corporation undertook a project at the request of NIOSH NTRC to help develop and apply an approach for identifying the center's contributions to the safety and health of workers who could be affected by the production, use, reuse, or disposal of engineered nanomaterials. This report describes the proposed method for gathering and organizing information about NTRC's operations and compiling information to capture the impact of its work. It also presents results from the RAND Corporation's application of the proposed method to a portion of NTRC's operations. For purposes of this pilot study and to test our model of NTRC operations, we limited our data collection concerning NIOSH outputs and stakeholder engagement to information and organizations related to nano–titanium dioxide and nano-silver.

In general, responsibility for capturing information about the efforts and products from research organizations, engaging with customers and partners, and collecting information about contributions to society will likely involve researchers, managers, and senior decisionmakers. Therefore, we expect this report to be of interest to a range of stakeholders, including NTRC senior executives, other NIOSH senior executives, and executives from other mission-oriented federal research and development agencies that either are planning to or are currently establishing processes to track impacts associated with their research and development activities. This report also should be of interest to researchers, program managers, and staff who are responsible for implementing, contributing to, or overseeing methods to assess the impact of their research efforts. In addition, the findings in this report will be of interest to researchers and workers who work with or are exposed to nanomaterials in occupational settings.

This report leverages past RAND research and contributes to ongoing work in research and development strategic planning and assessment, occupational safety and health, and emerging technologies and trends related to nanomaterials.

The RAND Safety and Justice Program

The research reported here was conducted in the RAND Safety and Justice Program, which addresses all aspects of public safety and the criminal justice system, including violence, policing, corrections, courts and criminal law, substance abuse, occupational safety, and public integrity. Program research is supported by government agencies, foundations, and the private sector.

This program is part of RAND Justice, Infrastructure, and Environment, a division of the RAND Corporation dedicated to improving policy and decisionmaking in a wide range of policy domains, including civil and criminal justice, infrastructure protection and homeland security, transportation and energy policy, and environmental and natural resource policy.

Questions or comments about this report should be sent to the project leader, Eric Landree (Eric_Landree@rand.org). For more information about the Safety and Justice Program, see www.rand.org/jie/research/safety-justice or contact the director at sj@rand.org.

Contents

Figures

Tables

Summary

In August 2014, the National Institute for Occupational Safety and Health (NIOSH) Nanotechnology Research Center (NTRC) asked the RAND Corporation to help develop and apply a method for assessing the center's contribution to improving the safety and health of workers who could be affected by the production, use, reuse, or disposal of the products of nanotechnology that are of greatest concern to workers, such as engineered nanomaterials. The purpose of the project was to develop a method that would help NTRC—and other NIOSH components—get beyond conventional bibliometric and patent analysis and closer to societal benefits or outcomes, in part by looking to the gray literature, professional events, and stakeholder outreach for supplemental evidence.

In general, an organization's activities and outputs are relatively straightforward to measure and track. However, it tends to be more difficult to measure and track an organization's contributions beyond those activities and outputs, such as how it is contributing to its strategic goals or desired societal outcomes. For a research organization like NIOSH that relies heavily on intermediate parties to achieve its mission of worker safety and health, this can be especially difficult. Given this challenge, RAND researchers worked with NTRC leadership to develop a description of the center's operations, referred to as a *logic model*, that characterizes NTRC's activities and outputs and how they are used by NTRC's customers and other intermediate parties to contribute to improved worker safety and health.

This report describes the method used to construct the NTRC logic model and includes insights and guidance for gathering and organizing information about NTRC's operations and their impact on or contributions to worker safety and health. RAND, in coordination with NTRC leadership, identified a portion of the organization to pilot this method and search for evidence of NTRC's activities and outputs that contribute to worker safety and health. For purposes of this pilot study, to test our model of the NTRC operations, we limited our data collection concerning NIOSH outputs and stakeholder engagement to information and organizations associated with nano–titanium dioxide (nano-TiO_2) and nano-silver (nano-Ag); this also allows us to assess the method's potential application to future, fuller assessments.

We identified a set of common categories of NTRC activities and outputs, as well as classes of stakeholders (spanning industrial, advocacy, governmental, research, educational, and training organizations) and workers, each of which makes use of NTRC's outputs in ways that have the potential to contribute to NIOSH's mission. Through a review of NIOSH documents, websites, and other publicly available information, we found examples of such use, suggesting that the proposed method can be used for the intended purpose.

We also identified, with input from NTRC leadership, a small number of external customers and intermediate parties with whom to discuss NTRC's outputs and services and how they are being used to affect worker safety and health. These discussions were used to verify and expand our initial logic model and to collect examples of NTRC contributions to worker safety and health related to engineered nanomaterials. Discussions with those customers and intermediate parties improved our understanding of how they learn about and receive products and services from NIOSH. Overall, the individuals we spoke with acknowledged NIOSH's expertise in occupational safety and health, and they were aware of NIOSH publications and bulletins related to nanomaterials. Within the scope of our pilot assessment, interviewees also identified examples of how NTRC is contributing to nanomaterial worker safety and health—for example, through changes in workplace practices in direct response to NIOSH publications or through direct engagement with NTRC field research teams. The NTRC customers and intermediate parties we spoke with also mentioned sharing NIOSH information and best practices among peers, competitors, and customers. In addition, they discussed how NIOSH publications are integrated into other types of documents or products, such as occupational safety training materials, and disseminated among communities of interest.

Our discussions also identified potential factors that might be inhibiting NIOSH's ability to achieve its desired outcomes. For instance, there is often not an explicit connection between the exposure to a particular nanomaterial, the health effect of that exposure, and the specific steps that should be taken in response to that exposure. In addition, the pace at which new nanomaterials are being developed and used by industry appears to exceed the pace of safety and health research and regulations, which can lead to outdated and insufficient rules. The lack of formal regulations may be limiting the use of on-site exposure monitoring, although premature regulation based on inadequate research and data may not be well received by NTRC customers and intermediate parties.

A more comprehensive review of NTRC across industry sectors, NIOSH-defined critical topic areas, and engineered nanomaterials or nanotechnologies is necessary to more fully characterize the breadth and scope of NTRC's success and barriers to achieving impact.

Acknowledgments

The authors wish to thank Charles Geraci, Laura Hodson, and Adrienne Eastlake from NIOSH for their cooperation and support throughout the course of this study. We also wish to thank those individuals outside of NIOSH who took the time to speak with us and share their views about NIOSH's nanotechnology-related outputs and how they are contributing to safer work environments.

We also are grateful for the support and counsel from RAND colleagues, particularly Brian Jackson and Tom LaTourrette, for their continued support. Finally, we would like to especially thank our reviewers, Philip Antón, RAND senior engineer currently on Intergovernmental Personnel Act assignment to the Department of Defense as the Deputy Director of the Acquisition Policy Analysis Center within the Office of the Undersecretary of Defense for Acquisition, Technology, and Logistics, and Caroline Wagner, associate professor and Ambassador Milton A. and Roslyn Z. Wolf Chair in International Affairs at Ohio State University. As always, the authors remain fully responsible for the content of this document.

Abbreviations

CDC	Centers for Disease Control and Prevention
C.F.R.	*Code of Federal Regulations*
CNT/F	carbon nanotubes or fibers
CPSC	Consumer Product Safety Commission
DHHS	U.S. Department of Health and Human Services
EPA	Environmental Protection Agency
FY	fiscal year
nano-Ag	nano-silver
nano-TiO$_2$	nano–titanium dioxide
NEAT	nanoparticle emission assessment technique
NIOSH	National Institute for Occupational Safety and Health
NIST	National Institute of Standards and Technology
NTRC	Nanotechnology Research Center
OSH	occupational safety and health
OSHA	Occupational Safety and Health Administration
PPE	personal protective equipment
RFI	Request for Information

CHAPTER ONE

Introduction

Overview of the National Institute for Occupational Safety and Health

The National Institute for Occupational Safety and Health (NIOSH) is the federal agency responsible for conducting research and making recommendations for preventing work-related injury and illness (Centers for Disease Control and Prevention [CDC], 2013a). NIOSH is part of the CDC within the U.S. Department of Health and Human Services (DHHS). The main legislative underpinnings of NIOSH are the Federal Mine Safety and Health Act of 1969 (or MSH Act; Pub. L. 91-173, amended by Pub. L. 95-164 in 1977) and the Occupational Safety and Health Act of 1970 (or OSH Act; Pub. L. 91-596).

The Occupational Safety and Health Administration (OSHA), which was also established as part of the OSH Act, is part of the U.S. Department of Labor and is responsible for developing and enforcing workplace safety and health regulations. NIOSH, in DHHS, was established to help ensure safe and healthful working conditions by providing research, information, education, and training in the occupational safety and health (OSH) field. NIOSH is typically described as a nonregulatory agency; however, it is directly responsible for several regulations. These include regulations related to the Coal Workers Health Surveillance Program, NIOSH grants and educational training programs, implementation of DHHS responsibilities under the Energy Employees Occupational Illness and Compensation Program Act, approval of respiratory protective equipment, investigations at places of employment for the Health Hazard Evaluation program and for occupational safety and health research, and implementation of the World Trade Center Health Program.[1]

NIOSH's staff consists of more than 1,200 employees with expertise in fields ranging from epidemiology, medicine, nursing, industrial hygiene, safety, psychology, chemistry, statistics, and economics, as well as various fields of engineering. According to the fiscal year (FY) 2015 Omnibus Appropriation and the FY 2015 CDC Operating Plan, the NIOSH budget was $335 million in FY 2015, which includes fund-

---

[1] More information about NIOSH-specific regulations and related parts of the *Code of Federal Regulations* (C.F.R.) can be found at CDC, 2013d.

ing for research, as well as for other programs and activities related to occupational safety and health.[2] NIOSH's primary organizing units consist of divisions, laboratories, and offices, shown in Figure 1.1. NIOSH has headquarters in Washington, D.C., and Atlanta, Georgia, with research laboratories and offices in Anchorage, Alaska; Cincinnati, Ohio; Denver, Colorado; Morgantown, West Virginia; Pittsburgh, Pennsylvania; and Spokane, Washington. The institute has matrixed its occupational safety and health activities across ten sector programs and 24 cross-sector programs that are distributed throughout the various divisions, laboratories, and offices. The NIOSH sector programs include Agriculture, Forestry, and Fishing; Construction; Healthcare

Figure 1.1
NIOSH Divisions, Laboratories, and Offices

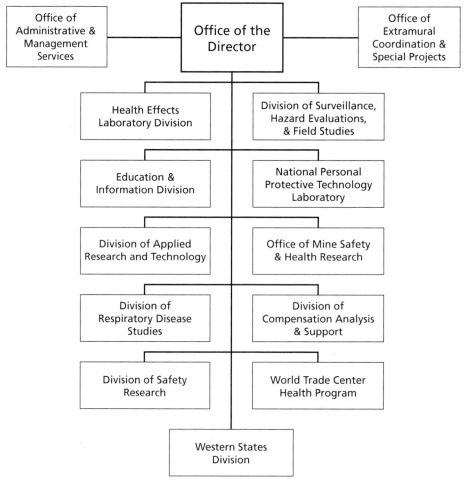

SOURCE: Adapted from CDC, 2015a.
RAND RR1108-1.1

---

[2]   For more details about the NIOSH budget, see CDC, 2015b, and Pub. L. 113-235, 2014.

and Social Assistance; Manufacturing; Mining; Oil and Gas Extraction; Public Safety; Services; Transportation, Warehousing, and Utilities; and Wholesale and Retail Trade, and the 24 cross-sector programs include such areas as Respiratory Disease, Economics, and Nanotechnology.[3] Research programs related to the sector and cross-sector programs are spread across the organizational units in NIOSH and thus are not a separate entity within the NIOSH organizational chart.[4]

Ten Years of NIOSH Nanotechnology Research

In 2004, NIOSH established the Nanotechnology Research Center (NTRC) as a virtual center to identify critical cross-sector issues concerning nanotechnology and nanomaterials; create a strategic plan for investigating these issues; coordinate the NIOSH research effort by engaging with scientists and engineers across NIOSH divisions, laboratories, and offices to develop research partnerships; and disseminate information related to nanotechnology. In addition to conducting research, NTRC works with industry and, in some cases, directly with workers. However, it also relies on other types of organizations, such as academic institutions and organized labor, industry, or trade associations, to reach out to workers on its behalf—for example, by developing measurement instruments, distributing educational materials, and delivering training on workplace safety. Like NIOSH, writ large, NTRC was set up to improve the safety and health of workers involved with engineered nanomaterials through conducting research, providing recommendations and workplace interventions, and supporting the training of occupational safety and health professionals to foster changes in workplace practices and reductions in workplace-related injuries, illnesses, and fatalities.

Over the past ten years, NTRC has helped direct the research efforts of more than 90 researchers, producing in excess of 900 scientific articles since 2004, and has engaged with industry, labor organizations, academic institutions, and other stakeholders on matters of worker safety and health; however, the extent to which those efforts have contributed to improvements in worker safety and health through changes in workplace practices and the reduction of workplace-related injuries, illnesses, and fatalities has not yet been established. According to the *National Nanotechnology Initiative Supplement to the President's 2016 Budget,* NIOSH's nanotechnology-related research budget in FY 2014 was $11 million, and it is estimated to remain the same for FY 2015 and FY 2016 (National Science and Technology Council, 2015, p. 22).

According to Williams and colleagues, "*Research impact* refers to the contribution of research activities to desired societal outcomes, such as improved health, environment, economic, and social conditions" (Williams et al., 2009, p. xi). There are several

---

[3] For a complete description of NIOSH's structure and NIOSH's sector and cross-sector programs, see CDC, 2013a, 2013c.

[4] The complete NIOSH organization chart is available at CDC, 2015a.

factors that complicate evaluating the impact of research efforts (Williams et al., 2009, p. 1). For instance, the lag between when a body of research is completed (and the results disseminated) and the time when the impact of that research is achieved can be on the order of decades, particularly in the case of fundamental research. In addition, the relationship between research efforts and impacts is typically diffuse and indirect, and it can be difficult to discern. For instance, multiple efforts or events (including other research efforts) may be needed to achieve a particular impact. Similarly, research findings can contribute to multiple different impacts, some well beyond their initial intent or domain. And a specific research result or finding may be passed between multiple entities, including other researchers, industries, or various intermediate parties before it ultimately contributes to a particular impact. Also, the lack of a program theory or conceptual model that describes how a research program achieves or contributes to desired outcomes or societal benefits makes it difficult to evaluate progress toward or contributions to those outcomes or benefits. Finally, the data for conducting evaluations can be difficult to locate, require intensive resources (e.g., time, money, manpower) to collect, and be subject to selection bias for positive impact.

As the number of industries and occupational settings that use nanotechnology and nanomaterials[5] expands, the possibility for workers to encounter these materials and to be exposed to them in the workplace will also likely increase. The expansion of these materials into increasingly diverse products, manufacturing processes, and workplace environments also presents a challenge for assessing NTRC's contributions to worker safety and health. In addition, trends in advanced manufacturing are redefining manufacturing and enabling access to sophisticated materials and capabilities to an increasing number of smaller companies. This diffusion of materials and capabilities to a growing number of companies and workers may complicate tracking the use of nanotechnologies and nanomaterials in the workplace, and may affect the implementation of good practices to reduce worker injuries, illnesses, or exposures. These trends are making it more difficult to understand where nanomaterials may be being used in occupational settings, which increases the challenges in understanding the potential risks and adds to the difficulty of assessing the adoption and efficacy of practices intended to reduce occupational injuries, illnesses, and exposure to nanotechnologies and nanomaterials.

Additionally, while it is relatively straightforward to track and measure an organization's activities and outputs, it is more difficult to track and measure its contributions to its strategic goals or desired societal benefits. For a research organization like

---

[5] For purposes of this report, the term *nanomaterials* is used generically to refer to a wide variety of nanoscale materials. It includes materials that are nanoscale in three dimensions (i.e., nanoparticles), two dimensions (i.e., nanofibers or nanorods whose diameter may be on the order of 100 nanometers or less, but could be microns or longer in length), or only one dimension (i.e., sheets of materials whose thickness is 100 nanometers or less, such as graphene). We use *engineered nanomaterial* to refer to both purposefully fabricated nanomaterials as well as nanoscale materials whose surfaces or stoichiometry have been engineered or functionalized with other materials to alter their physical, chemical, or electrical properties.

NIOSH that relies heavily on intermediate parties to achieve its mission of worker safety and health, this can be especially difficult. Given this challenge, the RAND Corporation worked with NTRC leadership to develop a description of the center's operations, referred to as a *logic model*, that characterizes NTRC's activities and outputs and how they are used by NTRC's customers and other intermediate parties to contribute to improved worker safety and health.

Problem Statement and Approach

In light of the challenges described above, assessing the contributions of NTRC's efforts to reduce occupational injuries, illnesses, and fatalities related to engineered nanomaterials requires a holistic approach that tracks the whole progression of those efforts—from developing the center's research agenda, to conducting research, to transferring and communicating results and guidance to key stakeholders, and to ultimately attaining changes in workplace practices or procedures that yield safety and health benefits.

In August 2014, RAND researchers undertook a project sponsored by NTRC to develop an approach for identifying the center's contributions to the NIOSH mission, specifically the safety and health of workers who could be affected by the production, use, reuse, or disposal of the products of nanotechnology that are of greatest concern to workers—that is, engineered nanomaterials—and then demonstrating that approach for a portion of the NTRC organization. This report presents the results of that project and outlines a method for gathering, organizing, and compiling information about NTRC's operations to capture the impact of its work, including its research and guidance. The purpose was to develop a method that would help NTRC (and other NIOSH components) move beyond bibliometric and patent analysis, and move closer to finding evidence of impact—such as changes in practice or procedures, or ideally examples of reductions in worker injuries, illnesses, fatalities, or exposures—by looking at other open literature and professional events, and by directly contacting stakeholders.

In brief, our approach consists of the following general steps:

1. Define the scope of the NTRC impact assessment.
2. Gather and review documents within the defined scope,[6] both to develop a preliminary logic model and to gather initial evidence of progress toward impact.
3. Produce a preliminary (or updated, if previous model is available) NTRC logic model consistent with the defined scope.
4. Identify and contact NTRC's stakeholders or a subset of stakeholders to inquire about their familiarity with and use of NTRC products (e.g., research findings, guidance documents, prototypes), both to further refine and finalize the pre-

---

[6] For purposes of this report, we use the term *documents* broadly to include NIOSH publications, as well as publicly available publications, memoranda, websites, and other sources of written, numeric, or pictorial information.

liminary (or updated) NTRC logic model and to gather additional evidence of progress toward impact.[7]

5.   Refine and finalize the NTRC logic model, document examples both of NTRC product use and of changes in stakeholders' practice or procedures, and present evidence of progress toward impact.

These five steps represent a process that can be applied to different portions of NTRC based on topic area, industry sector, or, as is this project, engineered nanomaterials of interest. The process could also be applied to portions of NTRC that have been assessed previously, to document further progress toward impact over time.

To pilot the method for potential application to future, fuller assessments, the RAND project team applied the steps to a portion of NTRC, focusing on the center's efforts regarding two engineered nanomaterials of interest—specifically, nano–titanium dioxide (nano-TiO_2) and nano–silver (nano-Ag).

Scope of Pilot Study

For Step 1 of our approach, we needed to select a portion of NTRC to pilot the proposed assessment method. NTRC's efforts apply to a wide range of industry sectors and NIOSH-defined critical topic areas, listed in Table 1.1. Working with NTRC leadership, we identified candidate nanomaterials that would have relevance across mul-

Table 1.1
Selection Criteria for Scoping the NTRC Pilot Study

Example Industry Sector	Critical Topic Area
• Coating (e.g., paints)[a, b] • Cosmetics (e.g., sunscreen)[a, b] • Construction (e.g., concrete)[b] • Services (e.g., cleaning, dry cleaning, food service)[a] • Electronics (e.g., semiconductor)[a] • Food additives[a, b] • Clothing, textiles, fabrics coating[a, b]	• Toxicity and internal dose • Risk assessment • Epidemiology and surveillance • Engineering controls and personal protective equipment (PPE) • Measurement methods • Exposure assessment • Fire and explosion safety • Recommendations and guidance • Global collaborations • Applications

SOURCE: Based on RAND analysis, with input from NTRC.

[a] This sector is an example of an identified product or manufacturing process that contains or uses nano-Ag or silver nanoparticles.

[b] This sector is an example of an identified product or manufacturing process that contains or uses nano-TiO_2.

---

[7]   Stakeholders include intermediate customers and end customers who make use of NTRC's products, services, and outputs. We discuss the different types of customers and other stakeholders in Chapter Two.

tiple industry sectors and topic areas, but that would not include the totality of the center (see Figure 1.2).

On that basis, we selected nano-Ag (also referred to as silver nanoparticles or AgNP) and nano-TiO$_2$ (also referred to as ultrafine TiO$_2$) as sufficiently representative engineered nanomaterials for the pilot effort. We used these two nanomaterials to limit our information-gathering to NIOSH documentation and to other available documentation that included references to either material and to the industry sectors, the NIOSH critical topic areas, or occupational safety and health concerns more broadly. We also used these two engineered nanomaterials to help us identify possible stakeholders to contact, which we discuss in more detail in Chapter Five. Both nanomaterials are relevant to multiple industry sectors and have been the focus of research related to multiple NIOSH critical topic areas (see Table 1.1). Moreover, in selecting these two materials, we were able to consider the applicability of the proposed approach both to a material that is well-established and to one that is garnering increased attention. For instance, nano-TiO$_2$ has applications in construction, cosmetics, and costing (among others) and has been a focus of NIOSH's research for several years. Alternatively, nano-Ag, which has been in commercial products for many years,[8] is gaining attention and interest for a growing number of commercial products because of its antibacterial applications, and it has more recently become a focus of NTRC's research efforts. In that regard, these two materials might be thought of as occupying different parts of the spectrum between an enduring commercialized nanomaterial and an

Figure 1.2
Selecting the Scope for the Pilot Effort

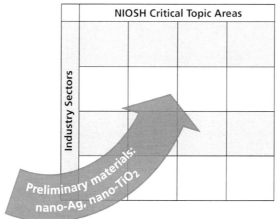

SOURCE: Based on RAND analysis, with input from NTRC.
RAND *RR1108-1.2*

---

[8] For more information on the history of silver nanoparticles, see Rauwel et al., 2015.

emerging nanomaterial. As we discuss in more detail in Chapter Five, we identified and contacted a small number of stakeholders within the scope of our pilot effort to collect feedback on the use and impact of NTRC's program efforts.

Organization of the Report

The report walks the reader through the five steps of our proposed method. Chapter Two describes our method for organizing information about impact, which consists largely of developing a logic model with which to trace the effects of NTRC's program efforts on worker safety and health. Chapters Three and Four describe our approach to compiling information to populate the model, as well as our initial findings, based largely on a content analysis of publicly available documents. Chapter Three focuses on program efforts, and Chapter Four focuses on program effects. Chapter Four also describes the various stakeholders that use NTRC's products and services, outlines a path by which those products and services are contributing to worker safety and health, and presents a preliminary version of the NTRC logic model. Chapter Five summarizes the findings from our discussions with NTRC stakeholders; presents a revised, final version of the NTRC logic model that incorporates information gleaned from those discussions; and shares insights from the pilot application that would be relevant to future assessments. Finally, Appendix A summarizes the steps described in this pilot project. The purpose of Appendix A is to provide NTRC—or potentially other NIOSH components—with a guide for collecting and updating information about how the center's efforts are furthering NIOSH's mission. Appendix B provides the NIOSH logic model, for reference, and Appendix C provides notional logic model worksheets.

CHAPTER TWO

Logic Models and Their Application to NTRC

This chapter includes a brief introduction to the concept of a logic model, related terminology, and its application to program evaluation. It also includes a brief discussion on the challenges of assessing the impact or outcomes from research programs. In addition, the chapter presents the NIOSH and NTRC mission and how it relates to our use of logic models.

Brief Introduction to Logic Models

A logic model is the primary tool with which we identify and communicate NTRC's contributions to the NIOSH mission. We chose to use logic models to frame our approach because of NIOSH's familiarity with logic models based on its previous program evaluation experience (CDC, 2013b). Here, we present some background on the use of logic models as we have applied it to NTRC.[1]

Logic models serve multiple purposes; most relevant to this project, they can help to identify a critical path or (often) multiple paths to achieving a set of desired outcomes that support an organization's mission. Constructing a logic model involves the development and description of the paths for how a program's or organization's efforts and the products of those efforts may plausibly contribute to its mission or desired effect. An important foundation regarding our use of logic models is that the process of constructing them is anchored to the organization's mission, or the societal benefit that is being pursued. Because of this focus on an organization's mission for assessing impact, logic models are not well-suited for capturing contributions to, or paths that lead to, impact beyond the scope of the organization's intended mission. For instance, a logic model for a research organization whose mission is to reduce occupational injuries, illnesses, and fatalities may not capture impacts that occur as a result of that research migrating beyond occupational safety and health.

---

[1] There are several sources of information on the theory and execution of program evaluation. Logic models represent only one approach. For a thorough review of the theory of program evaluation and methods for performing program evaluation of research and development programs, the authors recommend Shadish, Cook, and Leviton (1991) and Ruegg and Jordan (2007).

Applying a logic model compels mission-oriented research and development organizations to state explicitly the plausible intermediate steps for how their outputs or program efforts can be used or transformed by others to contribute to the desired effect (or mission). Once these plausible paths are described, they can then serve as a guide to help an organization identify where to look for evidence that supports its theory of how its efforts contribute to its mission or desired outcomes. Collected quantitative or qualitative evidence can then be used to support, convey, or demonstrate impact or contributions to its mission. The absence of evidence is also informative and may occur for several reasons. If an organization's theory of operation is not accurate, or it has not defined the plausible paths for how its program efforts can contribute to its mission, then it will be challenging (if not impossible) to find any evidence of impact. In other cases, and for research organizations in particular, a lack of evidence may suggest that there has not been enough time for the research findings and products to have contributed to desired impacts, as described in Chapter One. The presence or absence of evidence can then be used to help revise or update an organization's theory of operation, and perhaps better understand factors that are affecting its ability to achieve its intended mission.

Figure 2.1 provides a simple, blank logic model template that shows the key components and how they align relative to an organization's mission. While the amount of detail in logic models can vary, most include the following elements:[2]

- **Inputs** are the resources (e.g., staff, budget, research facilities) and information (e.g., strategic guidance, surveillance data, research requirements) that drive the day-to-day operations of an organization. We describe two different types of inputs, either production or planning. Production inputs refer to the monetary, human, or physical resources that are needed to support an organization's operation. Planning inputs include guidance documents, strategic plans, policies, or external data (e.g., medical surveillance data) that mandate, direct, or influence an organization's operations.
- **Activities** represent what an organization does on a daily basis. Depending on the size and complexity of the organization, the range of activities can be narrow or broad. In the case of the NTRC logic model, there are four general types of activities identified: conduct research; develop instrumentation, test equipment, protocols, and reference materials; conduct field assessments and monitor exposure; and provide policy, guidance, and recommendations and facilitate coordination among customers and partners.

---

[2]   A more comprehensive description of the elements of logic models is available in Williams et al. (2009), and additional discussions of applications can be found in Greenfield, Williams, and Eiseman (2006) and Greenfield, Willis, and LaTourrette (2012). For further background, we suggest, for example, McLaughlin and Jordan (1999); Taylor-Powell and Henert (2008); Wholey, Hatry, and Newcomer (2010); and W.K. Kellogg Foundation (2006).

Figure 2.1
Logic Model Template Highlighting Program Efforts and Effects

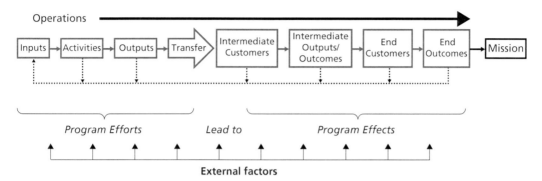

SOURCE: Adapted from Greenfield, Williams, and Eiseman (2006) and Williams et al. (2009).
RAND *RR1108-2.1*

- **Outputs** are the direct, tangible products (e.g., guidance documents, prototypes, scientific journal articles) that the organization's activities generate.
- **Customers** are the intended users or targets of an organization's outputs.
  - **Intermediate customers** are individuals or entities that use and transform an organization's outputs to produce intermediate products or intermediate outputs (see below) that would then be used by other intermediate customers or end customers. Examples of intermediate customers of NTRC's outputs include other research organizations, companies that manufacture nano-enabled products, agencies that produce regulations, industry associations, and other organized labor organizations.
  - **End customers** are individuals or entities that are the final target population that the organization seeks to affect. In the case of NTRC, the end customers are the workers, managers, or supervisors that encounter engineered nanomaterials in occupational settings.
- **Intermediate outputs** are the products or outputs created by an intermediate customer and can be used either by other intermediate customers or by end customers. Customers represent a subset of an organization's stakeholders, which might include partners with whom the organization undertakes various activities, as well as other interested parties.[3] In our discussions with stakeholders, we focused primarily on intermediate customers.

---

[3] We do not address the role of or engagement with partners as part of this report. Partners actively participate with an organization to generate that organization's products or outputs. The focus of this pilot effort was on organizations that received NTRC products. Therefore, while it is the case that some customers may also be partners, we do not discuss partners in detail. For more thorough descriptions of the potential role of partners, the authors recommend Greenfield, Williams, and Eiseman (2006) and Williams et al. (2009).

- **Outcomes** are changes in an environment or process that result from the use of an organization's outputs or the use of an intermediate customer's intermediate outputs; also referred to as *impacts*.
  - **Intermediate outcomes** can be changes in practice (e.g., the use of a new engineering control, changes in the handling of materials to avoid or reduce the risk of exposures) that lead to desired results or end outcomes.
  - **End outcomes** typically are societal, economic, or environmental benefits. End outcomes are closely connected to a program's strategic goals or stated mission.
- **External factors** are circumstances or events exogenous to the program that positively or negatively affect an organization's ability to achieve outcomes. External factors may affect any part of a program's operations from inputs to outcomes, including multiple areas simultaneously. Examples of external factors that may impact NIOSH's ability to achieve its intermediate and end outcomes may include significant changes in NIOSH funding or staff, new federal regulations, new (or changes to existing) manufacturing processes used by intermediate customers, or significant changes in demand for nano-enabled products or services.

An organization's *program efforts*, which consist of its inputs, activities, outputs, and transfer mechanisms, should lead to or contribute to its *program effects* or impact, which includes intermediate outputs, intermediate outcomes, and end outcomes. While there are specific increments or stages between inputs, activities, and outputs through to intermediate outputs and intermediate and end outcomes, the path is not necessarily linear. In many cases, information generated in a particular stage will result in feedback to an earlier stage, or serve as inputs to the start of the process. For example, notionally, research demonstrating that a particular line of investigation is not achievable or viable would generate information that would be fed back into inputs that would then redirect that effort to other possible areas of investigation. Another example is feedback from an end customer (i.e., worker) who is using a new piece of PPE that was developed by a manufacturer based on research findings (i.e., outputs) from NIOSH research activities. The end customer could suggest modifications to the design to improve its usability, and those modifications may enhance the equipment's use and adoption by other workers. End customers could also provide feedback to NIOSH that could inspire new research activities regarding performance or the form factor of the protective equipment, which could be transferred to intermediate customers to generate updated intermediate outputs. Feedback loops persist throughout the entire model, with information from each stage being generated and *ideally* fed back to previous stages to enhance the organization's potential contributions to its intermediate and end outcomes (i.e., to achieve greater impact).

NIOSH Mission and Connection to the NTRC Mission

Given the significance of an organization's mission to our logic model method, it is useful to present the NIOSH mission statement and describe how we have used it to drive the evaluation process for the NTRC program. According to the NIOSH website, its mission is as follows:

> NIOSH produces new scientific knowledge and provides practical solutions vital to reducing risks of injury and death in traditional industries, such as agriculture, construction, and mining. NIOSH also supports research to predict, prevent, and address emerging problems that arise from dramatic changes in the 21st Century workplace and workforce. NIOSH partners with diverse stakeholders to study how worker injuries, illnesses, and deaths occur. NIOSH scientists design, conduct, and support targeted research, both inside and outside the institute, and support the training of occupational health and safety professionals to build capacity and meet increasing needs for a new generation of skilled practitioners. NIOSH and its partners support U.S. economic strength and growth by moving research into practice through concrete and practical solutions, recommendations, and interventions for the building of a healthy, safe, and capable workforce. (CDC, 2013a)

A shorter version of the full mission statement is contained in the NIOSH logic model, which is provided for reference in Appendix B, and states that NIOSH's mission is "to provide national and world leadership to prevent work-related illnesses and injuries" (NIOSH, 2013b, p. 5).

NTRC does not have its own separate mission statement. Therefore, we modified the mission statement connected to the NIOSH logic model and used it as the mission to serve as the basis for our NTRC logic model. The modified mission statement that we used states that NTRC's mission is *to provide national and world leadership to prevent work-related illness and injuries resulting from exposures to nanomaterials.* We used this mission statement to anchor our identification and development of end outcomes and intermediate outcomes for NTRC, tracing back through intermediate customers, NTRC outputs, and so on. An example of a blank logic model worksheet similar to the one that was used to categorize and align the various pieces of information is shown in Table C.1 in Appendix C.

The modification of the NIOSH logic model mission statement to create an NTRC-specific mission is consistent with the program-level mission statements that were generated to develop logic models and compile evidence for the review of NIOSH by the National Academies from 2005 to 2008. All of the program-specific logic models and evidence packages developed for the National Academies review are available on NIOSH's website (CDC, 2013b).

CHAPTER THREE

Documenting NIOSH NTRC Program Efforts

In this chapter, we discuss information collected during our review of NIOSH documentation and open literature as part of Step 2 of our approach. We begin the process of developing an NTRC logic model as part of Step 3 by introducing the logic model elements that correspond to the NTRC program's efforts. This chapter describes inputs that drive the NTRC operations, the types of activities that NTRC is engaged in, and the corresponding outputs. We also include in this chapter a discussion of the transfer mechanisms that NTRC uses to transfer its outputs to various intermediate customers.

NTRC Inputs

In our approach, inputs occur as either production or planning inputs. Production inputs are the monetary, human, or physical resources that influence an organization's operations—for example, its budget or funding, staff, and laboratory equipment. Planning inputs include the data or information that influence, mandate, or direct the operations of an organization. They can include legislation, strategic guidance, information about stakeholder needs or workplace risks (e.g., workplace surveillance data), information about new materials, or new information about known materials or risks (e.g., scientific articles). Table 3.1 provides examples of the NTRC inputs that we identified in our document review.

NTRC Activities and Outputs

Our search for NTRC program efforts in the available documentation related to nano-TiO_2 and nano-Ag resulted in the four groups of activities shown in Table 3.2. The four categories of activities we identified are focused on conducting research; developing instrumentation, test equipment, protocols, and reference materials; conducting field assessments and exposure measurement on site; and developing policy, guidance, and recommendations. For each group, we found a corresponding collection of NTRC outputs, shown in the right column of the table.

Table 3.1
Preliminary List of NTRC Inputs

Inputs
Production
• Funding
• Staff
• Managerial support
• Laboratory and research facilities
Planning
• Budget, strategy, and planning documents
• Policies and plans
• Standards and guidance
• Needs or requests raised by stakeholders (i.e., partners, intermediate customers, and end customers)
• Risk assessment findings
• Scientific journal articles
• Animal and epidemiological studies

SOURCE: Based on RAND analysis of documents, with input from NTRC.

We generated the activities and outputs by looking for instances of nano-TiO$_2$ and nano-Ag in the documents collected. We modified the activities and outputs that we identified to make them more generally applicable to the broader NTRC. However, it is possible that a more comprehensive review of NTRC's operations—one that is not restricted to the two engineered nanomaterials selected as part of our initial scope—would produce additional activities and outputs.

While NIOSH is a research organization, the range of activities that NTRC is involved with and its corresponding outputs include more than just conducting research and producing journal articles and scientific publications about nanomaterials. There is a relationship between the different categories of activities listed in Table 3.2. For example, activities related to developing instrumentation, test equipment, protocols, and reference materials may be used to support activities associated with conducting research, and they may also contribute to activities related to conducting field assessments and monitoring exposure in occupational settings. All of these activities may then contribute to developing policy, NIOSH guidance documents, or recommendations that are captured in Current Intelligence Bulletins or NIOSH numbered documents. Each output can be transferred to its intermediate customers via a range of transfer mechanisms, which we discuss briefly in the next section. Consequently, the diverse range of activities and outputs suggests that multiple metrics and approaches would provide a more comprehensive summary of how NTRC is contributing to outcomes.

Table 3.2
Preliminary List of NTRC Activities and Outputs

Activities	Outputs
Conduct research	
• Research and evaluate the human health effects (e.g., pulmonary, respiratory, neuroimmune response, neurological) and toxicity associated with exposure to nanostructured materials (e.g., nanoparticles, nanotubes, nanofibers, and new forms of nanomaterials) • Research occupational exposures to nanostructured materials • Characterize the physical and chemical properties of nanostructured materials and products containing nanostructured materials • Characterize the transport mechanisms of nanostructured materials (e.g., aerosolized nanoparticles and nanowires) • Research and evaluate effectiveness of engineering controls and PPE for engineered nanomaterials	• Journal articles and scientific publications • Nanomaterials health and safety presentations
Develop instrumentation, test equipment, protocols, and reference materials	
• Develop methods and equipment to generate and characterize dispersed or aerosolized nanoparticles • Identify and develop nanoscale reference materials for calibrating measurement instruments • Evaluate diffusion charge-based sensors • Develop protocol for measuring nanomaterial mass and surface area in animal inhalation chambers • Develop and evaluate nano-aerosol surface area measurement methods • Develop procedures to test and evaluate the effectiveness of PPE	• Design for aerosolized nanoparticle generator to test exposures • Method for health hazard banding for nanostructured materials where potential toxicity is unknown • Technical input regarding nanostructured standard reference materials • Methods for measuring nanostructured materials' mass and surface area • Nanoparticle emission assessment technique (NEAT) • Draft standard for measuring mass and surface area of nanostructured materials
Conduct field assessments and monitor exposure	
• Conduct field research team site visits and exposure assessments • Assess occupational health risks associated with exposure to nanoscale materials • Analyze landscape of formulators and users of nanostructured materials • Contact and recruit companies for field assessments	• Site evaluation findings and reports • Survey of users and formulators of nanostructured materials
Provide policy, guidance, and recommendations	
• Chair and participate on standards bodies and associations • Respond to comments on Current Intelligence Bulletins	• Current Intelligence Bulletins • Recommended exposure limits • Recommended measurement methods • NIOSH numbered reports

SOURCE: Based on RAND analysis of documents, with input from NTRC.

NTRC Transfer

Table 3.3 shows examples of transfer mechanisms, and each either was captured through our review of NTRC and other documents or was inferred based on NTRC outputs or standard dissemination practices.

For many organizations, documenting evidence of contributions beyond outputs presents a significant challenge. For instance, it might be possible to monitor how often a particular presentation is made at scientific meetings or how many times a document is downloaded from the NIOSH website, but the exchange of information or knowledge that occurs through direct engagements with intermediate customers or workers is more difficult to track or quantify. Neither the time spent with stakeholders nor the number of new findings shared with stakeholders can fully reflect the potential value or contribution of this transfer mechanism for achieving outcomes. Nonetheless, the potential for this type of transfer to contribute to changes in workplace practices and enable intermediate and end outcomes is significant.[1] In addition, unlike other transfer mechanisms, direct engagement has the potential to impact final customers without having to pass through intermediate customers. For this reason, we call out the transfer that occurs through the NTRC field research teams as a separate mechanism for transferring NTRC outputs to both employers and workers that support the NIOSH mission, and we list it first among the transfer mechanisms identified.

The field research teams that engage with workers in occupational settings transfer a range of NTRC outputs. Depending on the circumstances, the teams may conduct on-site monitoring or provide recommendations on the use of engineering con-

Table 3.3
Preliminary List of NTRC Transfer Mechanisms

Transfer
• Conduct field research team site visits for face-to-face engagement with employers and workers at industries involved with the formulation or use of nanostructured materials
• Publish scientific findings in journals • Publish and disseminate NIOSH numbered reports • Present at scientific and OSH conferences and meetings • Sponsor or co-sponsor workshops on engineered nanomaterials • Demonstrate equipment • Update NIOSH blog

SOURCE: Based on RAND analysis of documents, with input from NTRC.

---

[1] The Howell, Silberglitt, and Norland (2003) report discusses the importance and value of on-site and direct engagement between the industry and researchers for finding effective solutions to industry-related problems. In addition, Section 2.6 of the *National Academies NIOSH Program Review: Health Hazard Evaluations* (CDC, 2007) discusses the transfer of information between NIOSH Health Hazard Evaluation response teams and staff working onsite at the workplace. Finally, Mitton et al. (2007) identifies face-to-face engagement with research users and research producers as being a key form of knowledge transfer and exchange.

trols, on changes to workplace practices, or on the use of PPE. There are also numerous other methods for transferring NTRC outputs to intermediate customers, such as publishing findings in scientific journals, presenting at scientific and OSH conferences, and demonstrating monitoring equipment at OSH conferences. Because these transfer mechanisms are focused primarily on the intermediate customer, we have grouped them together in Table 3.3, below the transfer that occurs from the field research teams. These different paths for the NTRC outputs will also be reflected in the preliminary NTRC logic model displayed at the end of Chapter Four.

From its literature review of knowledge transfer and exchange strategies for health care policy, Mitton et al. (2007, Table 4) identifies a compiled list of such strategies for the interchange of knowledge between research users and research producers. While there is not necessarily a one-to-one matching, there are similarities between the transfer mechanisms we identify in Table 3.3 and those described by Mitton et al. (2007). Specifically, those authors highlight face-to-face exchange, which is consistent with our characterization of the NTRC field research team's on-site engagement with employers and workers. In addition, publishing scientific findings in journals, publishing and disseminating NIOSH reports, and updating the NIOSH blog are consistent with Mitton et al. (2007)'s description of web-based information and electronic communications. Similarly, presenting at conferences and demonstrating equipment are also consistent with Mitton et al. (2007)'s category of interactive, multidisciplinary workshops. We have not tried to quantify which of these is more effective or more frequent for NTRC.

The next chapter discusses some examples of how NTRC program efforts that are specifically related to nano-TiO_2 and nano-Ag might contribute to outcomes that support the NIOSH mission.

CHAPTER FOUR

Documenting NIOSH NTRC Program Effects

In this chapter, we continue developing the NTRC logic model with Step 3 of our approach, and we describe the logic model elements that correspond to the NTRC program efforts, based on NIOSH and other available documents. We discuss the different types of intermediate customers and briefly describe the types of intermediate outputs, intermediate outcomes, end customers, and end outcomes. We also present the complete preliminary NTRC logic model that includes the elements described in this chapter and Chapter Three.

NTRC Intermediate Customers

A review of NIOSH and other documents, including two developed by RTI International for NIOSH (Sayes, 2013, 2014), suggested several categories and subcategories of intermediate customers, which we have listed in Table 4.1. For example, Sayes (2014) describes four distinct types of actors along the nanomaterial product life cycle: manufacturers, distributors, formulators, and users. That report goes on to identify companies that operate within a specific stage of the product life cycle and those that are involved in multiple stages of the nanomaterial product life cycle, extending from manufacturer to user.

In the following sections, we describe each category of intermediate customer and provide examples for the subcategories shown in Table 4.1.

Industry

Within the industry category, manufacturers are the companies that create or manufacture nanoscale materials, including such companies as QuantumSphere, Inc., which manufactures nano-Ag; DuPont, which manufactures TiO_2 particles on the order of hundreds of nanometers for various applications; and Cristal, which manufactures nano-TiO_2 on the order of tens of nanometers.

Distributors are companies that resell or distribute engineered nanomaterials to a broad range of customers. Sigma-Aldrich is an example of a distributor that sells materials, including nano-Ag and nano-TiO_2, that are used in the chemical, material, and life sciences.

Table 4.1
Preliminary List of NTRC Intermediate Customers

Intermediate Customers
Industry (establish policies/procedures) • Manufacturers of nanomaterials • Distributors of nanomaterials • Fabricators and formulators that use nanomaterials • Service industries that use or encounter nanomaterials • Manufacturers of instruments to monitor and manipulate nanomaterials
Advocacy • Business/industry associations • Law firms or legal organizations • Unions or other worker representatives • Other nongovernmental organizations • Other lobbyist groups
Government (international, federal, state, local) • Regulators • Government laboratories and researchers • Technology transition offices
Researchers and research institutions • Individual researchers • Academic research institutions • Other nongovernmental laboratories
Education and training • Universities • Training institutions • Trainers

SOURCE: Based on Sayes (2013, 2014) and RAND analysis of other documents, with input from NTRC.

Nanomaterials are incorporated or added into products in diverse ways. In some products, they may be added into another material or product in a suspension, and in others, they may constitute a discrete component or element of a larger product. Therefore, we expand Sayes (2014)'s original category of "formulators" to include both formulators and fabricators, reflecting the different ways in which engineered nanomaterials may be incorporated into products. In this context, formulators add nanoparticles to a matrix (which can be solid or liquid) in which the nanoparticles are held in suspension or distributed throughout the medium to provide enhanced or desirable properties. Examples of formulators that use nano-TiO_2 include some concrete, paint, and cosmetics companies, which use the materials to improve the performance of those products (e.g., better wear resistance, improved adsorption of ultraviolet wavelength light). Fabricators integrate nanomaterials into intermediate or finished products as a discrete element or component of a device or structure. Fabricators create products with engineered nanomaterials that are bound within the matrix to which they have been added (i.e., not free or unbound). An example of such a product is a nanomaterial whose surface has been coated or functionalized with different nanomaterials to create a sensing element for a detector whose electrical properties change in the presence of a particular target chemical or substance. Exposure to engineered nanomaterials depends on how the materials are handled and the manufacturing processes used and will vary between industry and products.

The fourth subcategory includes service industries that use products that contain engineered nanomaterials—for example, custodial companies that use cleaning products that contain nano-Ag and construction companies that use engineered nanomaterials that are integrated into other construction materials. This subcategory also includes the growing number of companies involved with the recovery, recycling, or disposal of products that contain engineered nanomaterials.

We also included a subcategory for the manufacturers of instruments to monitor and measure exposures to nanomaterials. Examples include TSI Incorporated and Dash Connector Technology, Inc., which have developed nanoparticle counters.

Advocacy

We use the term *advocacy* broadly to refer to groups or associations that might use NTRC outputs to create reports, pamphlets, or other such intermediate outputs to inform a target group or demographic, to advocate for a particular position, or to influence the views of policymakers, decisionmakers in industry, or others on a particular topic. The NanoBusiness Commercialization Association is an example of an organization that would fall under the advocacy category. While its members might include industries that manufacture, formulate, or distribute engineered nanomaterials, the NanoBusiness Commercialization Association advocates on behalf of its members to create an environment that is favorable to the commercialization of nanotechnologies and nanoscale materials. Other examples of industry-specific advocacy groups are the Silver Nanotechnology Working Group, the Titanium Dioxide Stewardship Council, and the American Chemistry Council Nanotechnology Panel.

Unions, worker representatives, or other organized labor would represent a different subcategory of advocacy. These organizations could potentially use NTRC outputs to advocate for changes in workplace conditions, changes to workplace practices, or additional training for workers.

Government (International, Federal, State, Local)

Government intermediate customers are the various international, federal, state, and local government agencies and offices that use NTRC's outputs. At the federal level, these include, for example, other government laboratories, such as the National Institute of Standards and Technology (NIST); government regulatory and research organizations, such as the Environmental Protection Agency (EPA) and OSHA; and other offices and programs within and across NIOSH.

Researchers and Research Institutions

The researchers and research institutions category refers to the individual researchers, universities, nongovernmental laboratories, think-tanks, and so on that might obtain NTRC research findings, scientific articles, or publications and use them to inform their current research and shape their research agendas. Among all the types of intermediate customers that we identified, those falling under the rubric of researcher and research institutions might be the easiest to substantiate—for example, through conventional bibliometric assessments or citation analysis. Insomuch as these types of customers make use of NTRC outputs in their own academic articles that are published in peer-reviewed, scientific, or other accessible journals, we would expect to find evidence of that use among their citations and references.

Education and Training

Intermediate customers involved with developing or providing education and training might also be involved in research, but, in this capacity, they might use NTRC outputs to produce training materials, create new engineering practices or procedures, and train individuals, as opposed to nanomaterials. Individuals could, for example, be trained in occupational or environmental health and safety practices and procedures related, in part or whole, directly or indirectly, to engineered nanomaterials. OSHA, some universities, and other organizations, such as some organized labor organizations, have or are affiliated with training or certification programs in occupational and environmental health and safety that might pertain to engineered nanomaterials. However, according to NTRC leadership, education and training in the handling and potential risks of engineered nanomaterials in the workplace also occur in laboratories that are training researchers and staff who are exposed to engineered nanomaterials through their work. As the number and variety of companies working with nanomaterials continues to expand, those NTRC customers who engage with education and training might be of increasing importance in helping NTRC connect with industry to increase the number of trained specialists who are implementing enhanced practices and procedures for the safe handling of engineered nanomaterials.

NTRC Intermediate Outputs and Intermediate Outcomes

The intermediate customers listed in Table 4.1 use a variety of NTRC outputs to produce a wide range of intermediate outputs that might contribute to changes in policies or practices in the workplace (i.e., intermediate outcomes). Based only on our initial review of NIOSH and other documents, we developed a preliminary list of NTRC intermediate outputs and corresponding intermediate outcomes (Table 4.2).

Table 4.2
Preliminary List of NTRC Intermediate Outputs and Intermediate Outcomes

Intermediate Outputs	Intermediate Outcomes
• Publications and research findings • Patents • OSHA Fact Sheet • OSHA recommended exposure limits • NIST Standard Reference Materials • Consumer Product Safety Commission risk assessment of products containing nanoparticles • Instrument for aerosol and hygiene sampling • Updates to 40 C.F.R. Part 721, "Significant New Uses of Chemical Substances" • Modified engineering controls and PPE • Training materials • Trained workers	• Acquisition of engineering controls and PPE in industrial processes • Use of NIST Standard Reference Materials • Use of NIOSH-developed measurement methods • Acquisition of monitoring and sampling equipment

SOURCE: Based on RAND analysis of documents, with input from NTRC.

NTRC End Customers and End Outcomes

The individuals that NIOSH and NTRC are trying to affect and who are most closely connected to NTRC's mission are the workers, supervisors, and managers and business owners who directly oversee those workers referred to in this logic model framework as end customers. Typically, as one gets further away from an organization's activities and outputs (i.e., program efforts) and closer to the organization's end customers and end outcomes (i.e., program effects), it becomes more difficult to distinguish how the organization's efforts have contributed to change as separate from the contributions of other organizations and actors. In some cases, it is possible to identify only a plausible causal link to an impact. For research organizations like NIOSH that rely heavily on intermediate customers (listed in Table 4.1) to achieve their missions, it can be especially difficult to document specific evidence that suggests impact. As discussed in more detail in Chapter One, this occurs for several reasons, including the fact that it can take many years for research outputs to move along the path to end outcomes. It might also be the case that the surveillance or monitoring necessary to document or measure changes along the path is missing or unobtainable; absent that capability, it might be difficult, if not impossible, to isolate a contribution. Table 4.3 lists the end customers most closely connected to the NTRC mission, as well as notional examples of intermediate outcomes and end outcomes that would support NTRC's mission.

The information compiled in our preliminary lists was used to develop a preliminary NIOSH NTRC logic model, shown in Figure 4.1. The logic model is a concept for how NTRC's *program efforts* (i.e., the left-hand side of the model that includes inputs, activities, outputs, and transfer) leads to desired *program effects* (i.e., intermediate customers, intermediate outputs, intermediate outcomes, end customers, and end outcomes).

Table 4.3
Preliminary List of NTRC End Customers and Notional Outcomes

End Customers	Intermediate Outcomes	End Outcomes
• Workers • Supervisors • Managers and business owners	• Adoption and use of engineering controls and PPE	• Reduction in work-related illnesses and injuries related to engineered nanomaterial exposures

SOURCE: Based on RAND analysis, with input from NIOSH NTRC.

There are some features within the preliminary NTRC logic model that emerged when the information contained in Tables 3.1, 3.2, 3.3, 4.1, 4.2, and 4.3 were translated into the logic model in Figure 4.1. As described in Chapter Three, NTRC activities associated with conducting research; developing instruments, test equipment, protocols, and reference materials; and conducting field assessments and monitoring exposure in the workplace are mutually supportive of and influence each other. This is highlighted in the logic model by the dashed arrows that connect these three boxes under the activities category. All of these activities contribute to the other main activity of NTRC, which involves providing policy, guidance, and recommendations. Consequently, there is an arrow that connects that activity box with the three activities listed above it. To the right of each major type of activity are examples of corresponding types of outputs that we could identify from the NIOSH and other available documentation.

From the outputs category, there are two major conduits for transferring the NTRC outputs. One is through the NTRC field research teams, who engage directly with workers in occupational settings to perform site assessments and monitor exposures, as well as develop recommendations for controlling exposures to engineered nanomaterials. A major feature of the NTRC field research teams is that they transfer NTRC outputs to the end customers without the necessity of working through intermediate customers and intermediate outputs. The other major conduit for transfer (also shown in Table 3.3 in Chapter Three) involves mechanisms for transferring NTRC outputs to the various types of intermediate customers.

Similarly, the logic model has the five categories of intermediate customers from Table 4.1. These intermediate customers generate a range of intermediate outputs (from Table 4.2), shown to the right of intermediate customers in Figure 4.1. Some intermediate outcomes are able to be realized through intermediate customers without needing to produce intermediate outputs—for instance, a manufacturer of engineered nanomaterials that implements a change in workplace practice in response to an NTRC recommendation. In addition, sharing of intermediate outputs and intermediate outcomes between intermediate customers can occur. This is highlighted with the feedback arrows from intermediate outputs and intermediate outcomes connecting back to intermediate customers.

Figure 4.1
Preliminary NIOSH NTRC Logic Model

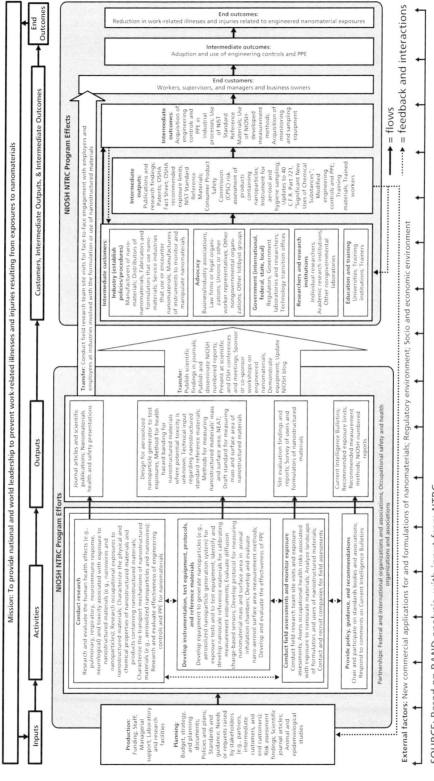

SOURCE: Based on RAND analysis, with input from NTRC.

RAND *RR1108-4.1*

Finally, intermediate customers may generate feedback that is used as an input to drive NTRC activities. Examples include requests for visits and risk assessments by the NTRC field research teams, as well as information about new products or research being done that may be relevant to nanomaterial OSH.

In the next chapter, we describe how we identified and selected a set of intermediate customers to contact for examples of how they were using NTRC outputs, and to help refine our NTRC logic model.

CHAPTER FIVE

Information About Intermediate Outputs and Outcomes from NIOSH NTRC Customers

In this chapter, we discuss criteria used to identify NTRC stakeholders to contact as part of Step 4 of our approach. We then review the information collected from intermediate customers about intermediate outputs, intermediate outcomes, and contributions toward end outcomes. We also present a revised logic model that incorporates information collected through this direct intermediate customer engagement.

NIOSH NTRC Customer Engagement

Using the information collected from the documents and discussions with NTRC leadership, we compiled the information shown in Tables 3.1 through 3.3 and Tables 4.1 through 4.3. We then used this information to construct a preliminary NTRC logic model, as shown in Figure 4.1, to illustrate the various paths by which NTRC's outputs might contribute to desired outcomes. Building on that foundation, we then identified a candidate set of intermediate customers for outreach, using the following three criteria:

- We looked for at least one company or organization for each category of intermediate customer listed in Table 4.1 and one that could serve as a surrogate for end customers, specifically workers, supervisors, and managers (see Table 4.3). It was thought that by contacting a smaller company, it might be possible to gain some insights about how NTRC's outputs influence end customers.
- We identified companies and organizations that either appeared in NIOSH documents or indicated in their own documents an awareness of or an association with NIOSH.
- We looked for companies or organizations that were connected with nano-TiO_2 and nano-Ag—for example, by production, use, reuse, recycling, or disposal of those materials.

On that basis and with feedback from NTRC leadership, RAND reached out to 11 intermediate customers and was able to schedule discussions with seven of them.[1] Each conversation lasted approximately 30 minutes. There was at least one representative for each of the five main categories of intermediate customer listed in Table 4.1.

We note that we were not attempting to reach out to all of the potential customers within the established scope of the project; rather, we were intending to reach out to a group of customers that, collectively, could enable us to test the feasibility of the approach and, to the extent possible, validate or suggest revisions to the preliminary NIOSH NTRC logic model. With regard to feasibility, we were seeking to demonstrate the possibility of gathering information on contributions to impact through direct engagement with intermediate customers.

Our discussions with intermediate customers generally focused on the following themes: the intermediate customer's general perceptions of NIOSH and NTRC and their outputs; how the customers become aware of or obtain NTRC outputs; how they use those outputs (e.g., research findings, recommendations, other publications, services); and how NTRC outputs affect their own products, services, or practices and contribute to impact or outcomes. We then extracted information from those conversations and identified elements that referred to transfer mechanisms, intermediate outputs, and intermediate and end outcomes.

The intermediate customers we contacted expressed familiarity with NIOSH, including NTRC. However, given that NTRC leadership provided feedback on our initial contact list, it is not surprising that our contacts expressed more than casual familiarity with NIOSH- and NTRC-related outputs. The intermediate customers identified the agency as having expertise in OSH and considered it to be a resource for trusted and unbiased information. Specifically, they mentioned the agency's expertise in respirators and its role in respirator certification. They identified NTRC as a potential source of support for on-site monitoring of engineered nanomaterials and as having constructive connections with industry. It was also mentioned that academic researchers who engaged with NIOSH were perceived as having greater credibility when they were approaching industries about research on OSH topics.

Speaking more directly to familiarity with NTRC, there was also wide awareness of NIOSH nanomaterial-related products, such as the Current Intelligence Bulletins on carbon nanotubes or fibers (CNT/F) and TiO_2. In addition, certain NIOSH guidance documents were viewed as helping establish research priorities to guide the research community in nanomaterial OSH. In general, these documents were well received.

---

[1] The conversations took place in February 2015.

Transfer

Our discussions uncovered a variety of transfer mechanisms. More than a few intermediate customers mentioned the field research teams' direct engagement with workers and industry (described in Chapter Three and highlighted in Table 3.3), which enables NIOSH to develop recommendations and protocols tailored to the recipient's specific needs. This transfer mechanism was identified as an important way for intermediate and end customers to become familiar with NIOSH outputs, and it is highlighted in Figure 4.1 with the single arrow at the top of Program Effects that goes directly from outputs to end customers. This mechanism was also identified as a way to provide NIOSH with knowledge about the on-site work environment. This is consistent with Mitton et al. (2007), which suggests that face-to-face encounters are critical to knowledge transfer and exchange.

The customers we spoke with mentioned several other transfer methods, including NIOSH Requests for Information (RFIs), which are published in the *Federal Register* and are a way for NIOSH to communicate OSH topics of interest to its customers. In addition, NTRC management and researchers directly engage with stakeholders as part of working groups, public-private focus groups, or partnerships. In another avenue for transferring information, NIOSH provides direct funding to specific intermediate customers to do research. Representatives of industry, government, and academia also mentioned that they refer inquiries on nanomaterial OSH from other (third) parties to NIOSH's website. Finally, at least one intermediate customer mentioned sharing NIOSH guidance and best practices directly with peers, competitors, and customers. This represents one type of evidence of transfer that would not be readily accessible and would be difficult to track without direct discussions with NTRC's intermediate customers.

One customer suggested that NIOSH might enhance its transfers to industry if it connected with industry through academic partners. The individual noted that with academia's emphases on research and on sharing information, those transfers might be more favorably received than direct transfers from NIOSH, which might be perceived as directive or regulatory in nature.

Intermediate Outputs

During our discussions, we discovered that several intermediate customers use or transform NTRC products and services to create their own products, documents, or services (i.e., intermediate outputs). For example, more than one intermediate customer mentioned developing training materials and conducting training sessions with organized labor unions using NTRC-related research findings. Another training course that was developed for safety and health practitioners with support from OSHA funding leveraged NIOSH findings. The second course, which included NTRC information on engineered nanomaterials, was accessed on the Internet more than 35,000 times.

Another example of an intermediate output was a data repository, created for workers and unions and informed by NTRC outputs, that listed construction products purported to be nano-enabled. Another intermediate customer mentioned requesting a health hazard evaluation to look at nano-enabled construction products, which led to a NIOSH evaluation at a training school. One intermediate customer also developed and distributed a survey (based on NTRC outputs) to workers to assess their awareness of engineered nanomaterials and nano-enabled products.

There were also examples of an intermediate customer providing intermediate outputs to a different intermediate customer. This exchange of information could occur either within a certain subcategory of intermediate customer (e.g., sharing NIOSH recommendations between industries dealing with the same material) or across intermediate customer subcategories. For example, an intermediate customer that was a federal organization mentioned that companies had sent it chemical notices that included NIOSH data generated from site evaluations.

Edging closer to an intermediate outcome, we learned of a company that modified its in-house recommended exposure limits for engineered nanomaterials based on NIOSH recommendations. NIOSH outputs also appear to have informed the manufacture of monitoring equipment, which is largely being used by researchers at academic institutions to quantitatively measure air samples for nanoparticles. And at least one intermediate customer mentioned that NIOSH outputs are shared in the research community to build awareness, facilitate engagement with industry, generate new research collaborations, and evaluate laboratory practices for handling engineered nanomaterials.

In addition, one intermediate customer who works with industry described circulating NTRC outputs to other associated organizations to inform, develop feedback, and motivate responses to NIOSH-published RFIs. In developing their RFI responses, the organizations, at a minimum, would have reviewed their own practices for handling the nanomaterial in question for compliance with current material safety data sheets. Finally, more than a few intermediate customers prepared reports, strategic research documents, or briefings or conducted demonstrations that leveraged or were informed by NIOSH nanotechnology-related research and outputs; these were then further disseminated through various scientific and OSH-related conferences and meetings.

Our discussions indicated a need for refinements—including additions and modifications—to the preliminary NIOSH NTRC logic model. In particular, the discussions provided additional information about intermediate outputs that allowed us to break them out and align them to their corresponding intermediate customers. In Figure 4.1, all of the intermediate outputs are under a single heading, but in the updated portions of the logic model presented in Figure 5.1, the intermediate outputs are now in groups and are aligned with their corresponding intermediate customer groups. (The differences from Figure 4.1 are highlighted in red.)

Figure 5.1
Proposed Refinements to the Preliminary Logic Model's Intermediate Customers and Intermediate Outputs

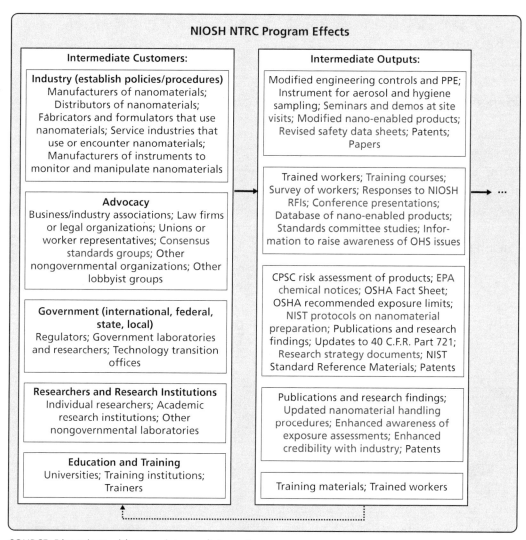

SOURCE: Discussions with seven intermediate customers.
RAND RR1108-5.1

Intermediate and End Outcomes

Our conversations left us with fewer specific examples of intermediate or end outcomes compared with the number of examples of intermediate outputs. However, some intermediate customers did mention changes in workplace or on-site practices or procedures that occurred in response to NIOSH outputs. In many of those cases, they mentioned that this change in practice was a result of the NTRC field research teams' direct engagement with the intermediate customers. We also learned of changes in on-site practices or procedures based on NIOSH information or outputs that had been shared through other intermediate customers. One specific, if circuitous, example was of a manufacturer of a nano-enabled product changing its manufacturing processes partly because of feedback that it received from a labor union that was informed by work from NIOSH.

Evidence of Impact and Revised NTRC Logic Model

The above descriptions of intermediate outputs and, to a lesser extent, intermediate outcomes suggested that NTRC is making at least some progress toward and contributing to NIOSH's mission. We note, for example, the repeated references to the work of field teams as conduits for reaching intermediate and end outcomes. Several intermediate customers emphasized the role of the NTRC field research teams in contributing to changes in workplace practices and procedures, introducing controls, and conducting on-site monitoring and assessments. However, given the limited scope of our pilot effort and the relatively small number of intermediate customers that we spoke with, a more comprehensive review of NTRC across industry sectors, critical topic areas, and engineered nanomaterials or nanotechnologies would be necessary to more fully characterize the breadth and scope of the program's impact.

At the same time, our conversations with intermediate customers also suggested the need to refine the preliminary NIOSH NTRC logic model. In addition to the changes shown in Figure 5.1, we also captured two additional points regarding NTRC's activities and transfer methods. More than a few customers mentioned the important function that NIOSH serves in bringing interested parties together on the topic of OSH for engineered nanomaterials. This activity was not identified previously, during our review of the literature, and is reflected in the revised model in Figure 5.2 as an NTRC activity (in red). In particular, we expanded the activities related to providing policy, guidance, and recommendations to include facilitating the coordination of information among interested partners and customers.

In addition, customers we spoke with also described direct engagement with NTRC senior staff and researchers as an important conduit for learning about and transferring information about NTRC outputs. Several customers mentioned that they would learn about NIOSH and NTRC outputs through these direct engagements, either as part of mutual participation on committees or through personal correspondence, rather than through formal publications or the NIOSH website. As noted, feedback from NTRC leadership in selecting our contacts might have led us to speak with especially engaged customers; nonetheless, the conversations suggested a significant path for transferring information about NIOSH's outputs to intermediate customers that we did not capture during the initial literature review. To capture this path in the revised logic model, we added "directed engagement" to the transfer arrow (see Figure 5.2).

Figure 5.2
NIOSH NTRC Logic Model, with Revisions

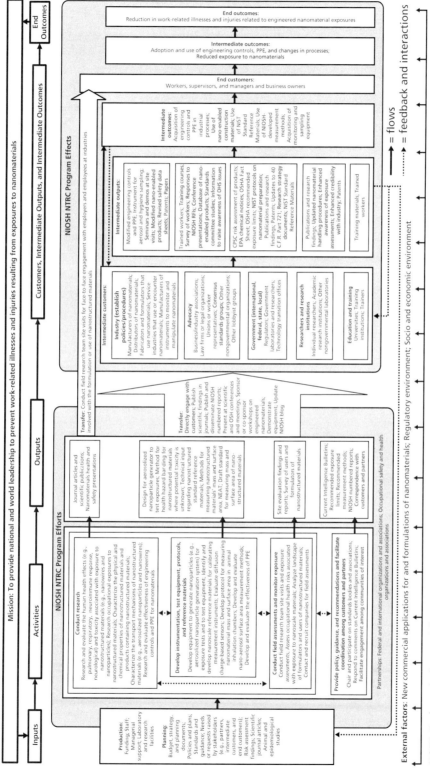

NOTE: Red text indicates differences from Figure 4.1.

RAND RR1108-5.2

Other Topics Raised by Intermediate Customers

During our discussions, several individuals acknowledged that NIOSH supports multiple intermediate customers (e.g., workers, industry, regulators, and researchers), all with different interests and needs. This differentiation is reflected in the NTRC logic model (see Table 3.2 and Figure 5.2), which highlights the different types of activities (i.e., conduct research; develop instruments, test equipment, protocols, and reference materials; conduct field assessments and monitor exposure; and provide policy, guidance, and recommendations and facilitate coordination among customers and partners) that result in different types of NTRC outputs. In the logic model, we also differentiate two paths for transfer. One is a direct transfer of NTRC outputs to workers via NTRC field research teams. The other is a collection of multiple transfer mechanisms that potentially provide information to various intermediate customers.

In addition to providing insights on how NTRC program efforts contribute to program effects, our conversations with intermediate customers also raised potential concerns about factors that might be inhibiting NIOSH's ability to achieve its desired outcomes.

Some customers raised concerns about what they described as a "knowledge gap" between exposure, toxicological response, and potential health outcomes. They gave three specific examples: a lack of standardized metrics for measuring nanomaterial exposures, a lack of specific personal exposure limits, and a lack of information about the potential effects of exposures to a wide range of engineered nanomaterials. For most engineered nanomaterials today, there is no clear, explicit connection between the exposure to a particular nanomaterial, the health effect of that exposure, and specific steps that should be taken in response to that exposure. This is in contrast to most chemical substances, where the personal exposure limit, the health consequences for exceeding that limit, and the necessary actions in response to an exposure are better understood. One customer suggested establishing incentives for monitoring exposures in the workplace. Another option would be to focus research efforts on some of the identified gaps.

Another customer mentioned that small businesses lack awareness of NIOSH or OSH issues and might have limited resources for on-site monitoring and assessments. The customer suggested that NIOSH could mitigate this issue partly by a more aggressive outreach effort so that its expertise and services are more widely known by the small businesses and industries that lack the resources for dedicated or in-house OSH services.

Customers also raised the concern that industry is moving faster than safety and health research and faster than regulations, which can lead to outdated rules and regulations. One customer noted that a lack of formal regulations might contribute to a lack of on-site exposure monitoring by the company. However, a regulation based on inadequate research and data may not be well received. Thus, it was suggested that regulations address the difficult balance between the most up-to-date research findings, occupational exposure risks, and impact on industry.

In addition, more than a couple of the intermediate customers we spoke with described the NTRC field research team as a valuable asset in monitoring workplace exposure to engineered nanomaterials and commented that they seemed to be in high demand. At least one customer posited that the field team's engagements are limited by resources (e.g., staff, budget) and, in some cases, lack of support from host companies. At least one customer also suggested that devoting additional resources to the field research team could contribute to better OSH outcomes.

Our discussions also revealed that the amount of time NIOSH takes to review and publish reports or conference proceedings was a concern to intermediate customers. It was suggested that, while the research findings and guidance documents are sound and accurate when published, the rapid pace of change in the industry (e.g., updated manufacturing processes, introduction of new materials) means that these documents may not be current or as relevant by the time they are released. In addition, although NTRC is perceived as conducting high-quality research and typically producing relevant products, including training materials for OSH professionals, at least one intermediate customer expressed interest in having NIOSH develop training materials targeted directly at educating workers on engineered nanomaterials.

Observations on the Pilot Engagement with Stakeholders and Next Steps

In conducting our discussions with intermediate customers, we made several observations that we felt would be relevant should NTRC pursue this type of assessment beyond the scope of this pilot effort. Specifically, we observed that different organizations interpret and understand the terms *outcomes* and *impact* differently from one another. When we asked intermediate customers to describe examples of how NIOSH has contributed to outcomes, some described new documents or proposals; others viewed outcomes in terms of manufactured products or regulations. Only occasionally did they view outcomes in terms of improvements in worker safety or health, without prompting. It was useful to learn about how different intermediate and end customers interpreted and understood NIOSH's mission, and how they viewed their role in achieving a desired impact or benefit.

Also, directly engaging with NIOSH stakeholders was critical for assessing, modifying, and refining the NIOSH NTRC logic model. As this pilot study indicated, the theory of how NIOSH's program efforts would contribute to desired outcomes was not inaccurate, but it was refined with information gained through the stakeholder discussions. Our discussions with NTRC intermediate customers provided context and details about how NTRC's outputs are being shared and circulated among intermediate customers and contributing to intermediate outcomes. The discussions also provided a means for identifying additional customers—through a snowball effect—who could have been contacted for further insight.

Initially, we focused on nano-TiO$_2$ and nano-Ag because they represented an enduring commercialized nanomaterial and an emerging nanomaterial. However, through the course of our pilot effort, there did not appear to be a difference between NTRC's progress toward outcomes for either engineered nanomaterial. We cannot state whether lack of evidence of intermediate and especially end outcomes was a reflection of the inherent difficulty of finding such evidence or of the small number of intermediate customers in our pool of contact.

Nonetheless, the method outlined in this report does provide NTRC (or, with minor modifications, other parts of NIOSH) with a guide for collecting, organizing, and assessing information related to NTRC's program efforts and how they are contributing to NIOSH's desired outcome of reducing injuries, illnesses, and fatalities associated with occupational exposure to engineered nanomaterials.

Regarding next steps, there are several options for how NTRC could proceed. This report described a process to assist NTRC with collecting information about its contributions to outcomes (also described in Appendix A), and then demonstrated that process for a portion of the center. One potential next step would be for NTRC to use the logic model developed here as a starting point to compile additional information about contributions to outcomes for different materials, critical topics areas, or industry sectors. Another potential next step would be to use this report as a point of departure to develop a more comprehensive set of metrics to help drive the identification and collection of data for assessing contributions to outcomes. Each component of the NTRC logic model suggests possible metrics, whether they are annual measures to track activity, outputs, and transfers; intermediate measures to monitor progress toward intermediate outcomes; or strategic measures to track progress toward end outcomes. Once metrics have been defined for each component of the logic model (i.e., from inputs to outcomes), the next step would involve identifying and cataloging data that are already available, data that currently exist but that are not used or available to NIOSH, and data that do not exist or are not currently collected but that would be desirable for tracking NTRC's contributions to outcomes. These metrics and data could be used to drive the development of new data collection methods or tools, or could drive new partnerships to help make more data available to NIOSH for tracking contributions to outcomes. This type of information could be used to help provide insights into which NTRC outputs are more successful at contributing to outcomes, as well as what factors may be affecting that success. That information could then be used to inform NTRC's pursuit of support for various outputs and transfer mechanisms.

Another possibility would be to systematically collect descriptions of the expectations or requirements from representative organizations for each of the subcategories of intermediate customers identified in Table 4.1 and end customers described in the NTRC logic model. This information could then potentially be used to develop metrics to help track whether and how adequately those expectations or requirements are being met. As more data are captured, and through continued advances in information technology systems, a future goal could be to integrate metrics and data collection systems into a research and development program planning and tracking system that could be used to help provide better situational awareness of how past and current research programs are contributing to desired outcomes. Finally, the logic model method developed here could also be used to help drive NTRC strategic planning to help ensure that strategic goals align with desired end outcomes, that intermediate goals align with intermediate outcomes, and that annual goals are consistent with NTRC activities and outputs.

Guide for Collecting Evidence of Contributions to NIOSH NTRC Outcomes

In this appendix, we provide a guide for evaluating the impact of NTRC's research based on the experience from this pilot project. The appendix is written as a standalone document that focuses on the method and steps that were demonstrated in the main body of the report. It is provided here without the additional information that was collected as part of the pilot study to serve as a reference for individuals who are applying this method to other portions of NTRC. The five steps of the assessment process are as follows:

1. Define the scope of the NTRC impact assessment.
2. Gather and review documents within the defined scope, both to develop a preliminary logic model and to gather initial evidence of progress toward impact.
3. Update the existing NTRC logic model (or generate a preliminary model if no previous model is available), consistent with the defined scope.
4. Identify and contact NTRC's stakeholders or a subset of stakeholders to inquire about their familiarity with and use of NTRC products (e.g., research findings, guidance documents, prototypes), both to further refine and finalize the preliminary (or updated) NTRC logic model and to gather additional evidence of progress toward impact.
5. Refine and finalize the NTRC logic model, document examples both of NTRC product use and of changes in stakeholders' practice or procedures, and present evidence of progress toward impact.

Note that the impact assessment is not a one-time effort; rather, it is designed to be iterative and repeated as necessary or appropriate—for example, whenever research priorities or funding situations change. The reassessment could be done annually, or more or less frequently depending, for example, on the timing of change.

We describe in detail each step of the assessment process below.

Define the Scope of the Assessment

The first step is to determine the scope of the assessment. Research at NTRC spans a wide range of materials (e.g., ultrafine-TiO_2, silver nanoparticles, CNT/F), industries (e.g., coatings, cosmetics, construction), and NIOSH-defined critical topic areas (e.g., toxicity and internal dose, risk assessment, and epidemiology and surveillance). The scope can be based on any one or a combination of these categories. While the method we describe may be applied to the entire NTRC, given the diverse range of industry sectors, materials, critical topic areas, and intermediate and end customers related to nanotechnology, reviewing the entire NTRC at once would require more effort and resources than reviewing a portion of NTRC. Therefore, the available resources (e.g., staff and researcher time and availability, budget, opportunity costs) should be taken into consideration when deciding the scope. Table A.1 shows a few potential selection criteria to consider.

As mentioned, the scope of the assessment might be limited to a single industry sector, a single critical topic area, or a single nanotechnology or nanomaterial. The scope might be narrowed or focused further by looking at the intersection of two or more of these criteria, as shown in Figure A.1. Some considerations include the size of industry sectors, amount of NTRC research on a particular nanotechnology or nano-material, and critical topic areas. Evaluations of large industry sectors, widely used nanomaterials, and critical topic areas that occupy a large share of the NTRC research portfolio might yield more examples of contributions to impact than narrower evaluations, but NTRC might need to allocate more resources to conduct the review.

Table A.1
Examples of Selection Criteria for Scoping NTRC Assessment

Example Industry Sector	Critical Topic Area	Nanotechnology or Nanomaterial
• Coating (e.g., paints) • Cosmetics (e.g., sunscreen) • Construction (e.g., concrete) • Services (e.g., cleaning, dry cleaning, food service) • Electronics (e.g., semiconductor) • Food additives • Clothing, textiles, fabrics coating	• Toxicity and internal dose • Risk assessment • Epidemiology and surveillance • Engineering controls and PPE • Measurement methods • Exposure assessment • Fire and explosion safety • Recommendations and guidance • Global collaborations • Applications	• Nano-TiO_2 • Nano-Ag • CNT/F

SOURCE: Based on RAND analysis, with input from NTRC.

Figure A.1
Venn Diagram of Criteria for Scoping the NTRC Assessment

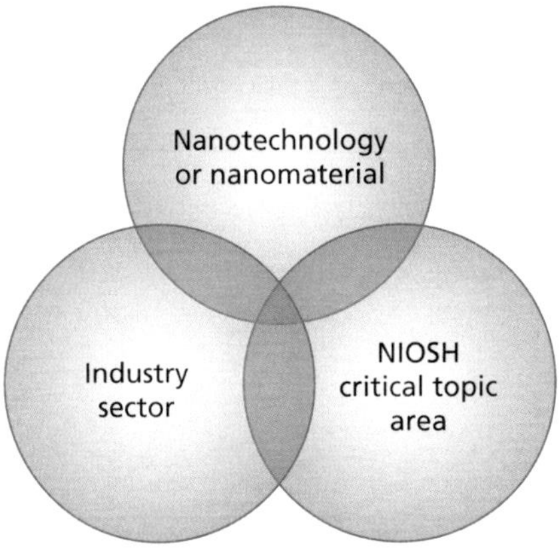

SOURCE: Based on RAND analysis, with input from NTRC.
RAND *RR1108-A.1*

Gather and Review Documents Within the Defined Scope

After defining the scope, Step 2 is to gather and review information on NTRC research and its impact. This should include reviewing the most recent NTRC logic model (shown in Figure A.2) and any other relevant NIOSH logic models to serve as a point of departure for the assessment. The *logic model* is a tool for organizing and conceptualizing the connection between NTRC research and impact on OSH.[1]

A generic logic model is typically composed of the following elements:

- **Inputs** are the resources (e.g., staff, budget, research facilities) and information (e.g., strategic guidance, surveillance data, research requirements) that drive the day-to-day operations of an organization. In the NTRC logic model, we have two types of inputs, either production or planning. Production inputs refer to the monetary, human, or physical resources that are needed to support an organization's operation. Planning inputs include guidance documents, strategic plans, policies, or external data (e.g., medical surveillance data) that mandate, direct, or influence an organization's operations.
- **Activities** represent what an organization does on a daily basis. Depending on the size and complexity of the organization, the range of activities can be narrow or

---

[1] A more comprehensive description of the elements of the logic model is available in Williams et al. (2009), and additional discussions of applications can be found in Greenfield, Williams, and Eiseman (2006) and Greenfield, Willis, and LaTourrette (2012). For further background, we suggest, for example, McLaughlin and Jordan (1999); Taylor-Powell and Henert (2008); Wholey, Hatry, and Newcomer (2010); and W.K. Kellogg Foundation (2006).

Figure A.2
NIOSH NTRC Logic Model

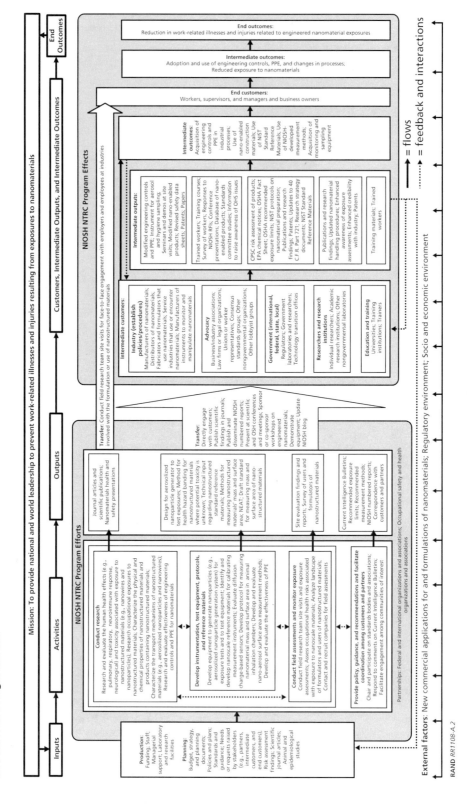

RAND RR1108-A.2

broad. In the case of the NTRC logic model, there are four general types of activities identified: conduct research; develop instrumentation, test equipment, protocols, and reference materials; conduct field assessments and monitor exposure; and provide policy, guidance, and recommendations and facilitate coordination among customers and partners.

- **Outputs** are the direct, tangible products (e.g., guidance documents, prototypes, scientific journal articles) that the organization's activities generate.
- **Customers** are the intended users or targets of an organization's outputs.
  - **Intermediate customers** are individuals or entities that use and transform an organization's outputs to produce intermediate products or intermediate outputs (see below) that would then be used by other intermediate customers or end customers. Examples of intermediate customers of NTRC's outputs include other research organizations, companies that manufacture nano-enabled products, agencies that produce regulations, industry associations, and other organized labor organizations.
  - **End customers** are individuals or entities that are the final target population that the organization seeks to affect. In the case of NTRC, the end customers are the workers, managers, or supervisors that encounter engineered nanomaterials in occupational settings.
- **Intermediate outputs** are the products or outputs created by an intermediate customer and can be used either by other intermediate customers or by end customers. Customers represent a subset of an organization's stakeholders, which might include partners with whom the organization undertakes various activities, as well as other interested parties.[2] In our discussions with stakeholders, we focused primarily on intermediate customers.
- **Outcomes** are changes in an environment or process that result from the use of an organization's outputs or the use of an intermediate customer's intermediate outputs; also referred to as *impacts*.
  - **Intermediate outcomes** can be changes in practice (e.g., the use of a new engineering control, changes in the handling of materials to avoid or reduce the risk of exposures) that lead to desired results or end outcomes.
  - **End outcomes** typically are societal, economic, or environmental benefits. End outcomes are closely connected to a program's strategic goals or stated mission.
- **External factors** are circumstances or events exogenous to the program that positively or negatively affect an organization's ability to achieve outcomes.

---

[2] Partners actively participate with an organization to generate that organization's products or outputs. The focus of this pilot effort was on organizations that received NTRC products. Therefore, while it is the case that some customers may also be partners, we do not discuss partners in detail. For more thorough descriptions of the potential role of partners, the authors recommend Greenfield, Williams, and Eiseman (2006) and Williams et al. (2009).

In addition, if the portion of the NTRC under assessment has significant connections to other NIOSH programs, it could be useful to review other NIOSH logic models, such as those generated for the National Academies' external review of NIOSH (CDC, 2013b). A review of the NTRC logic model and other NIOSH logic models, as appropriate, could help NTRC confirm that its operations align with its goals and objectives and with those of the larger agency. A review might also allow NTRC to ask whether any strategic changes within the center or changes in direction, resources, or effort need to be reflected in a revised logic model. This step will also help guide and inform the collection of relevant documents and identify partners and customers that should be contacted, as described in the next steps.

Update the Logic Model

Step 3 in the process is to update the NTRC logic model (or generate a new preliminary logic model) consistent with the defined scope.

After reviewing the most recent logic model, it is necessary to gather and review information on NTRC research and its impact. Sources of information should include NIOSH documents[3]—such as the Current Intelligence Bulletins, the NTRC website (for example, CDC, 2014), and other NIOSH-related research publications, including those published externally—as well as other relevant non-NIOSH documents.

This step also should include discussions with NIOSH managers, researchers, and staff affiliated with NTRC, within the scope of the review. The discussion should focus on NTRC activities and outputs and on identifying key customers and partners. Information pertaining to intermediate outputs or outcomes should also be identified, captured, and transferred to a logic model worksheet, shown schematically in Figure A.3.

The worksheet is another tool for compiling, reviewing, and aligning information relevant to conveying impact. Each column of the worksheets corresponds to different logic model elements described in the previous step. Once the worksheet is filled out, one can review it to look for commonalities among the items listed underneath each column to ensure that they are all of the same type. For example, one can check to ensure that everything under the Activities column contains only examples of actions or descriptions of actions (i.e., verbs) that NTRC has taken or is currently taking (i.e., are the contents of the cells labeled (a) and (g) in Figure A.3 of the same type?). Similarly, one can check to make sure that everything under the Outputs column includes only objects or things (nouns) that would result from an action (i.e., are the contents of the cells labeled (b) and (j) in Figure A.3 of the same type?). The process of vertical inspection can serve at least two purposes. It can be used to identify and correct mis-

---

[3]   As noted at the outset of this report, we use the term *documents* broadly, to include publications, memoranda, websites, and other sources of written, numeric, or pictorial information.

Figure A.3
Notional Logic Model Worksheet, with Annotation

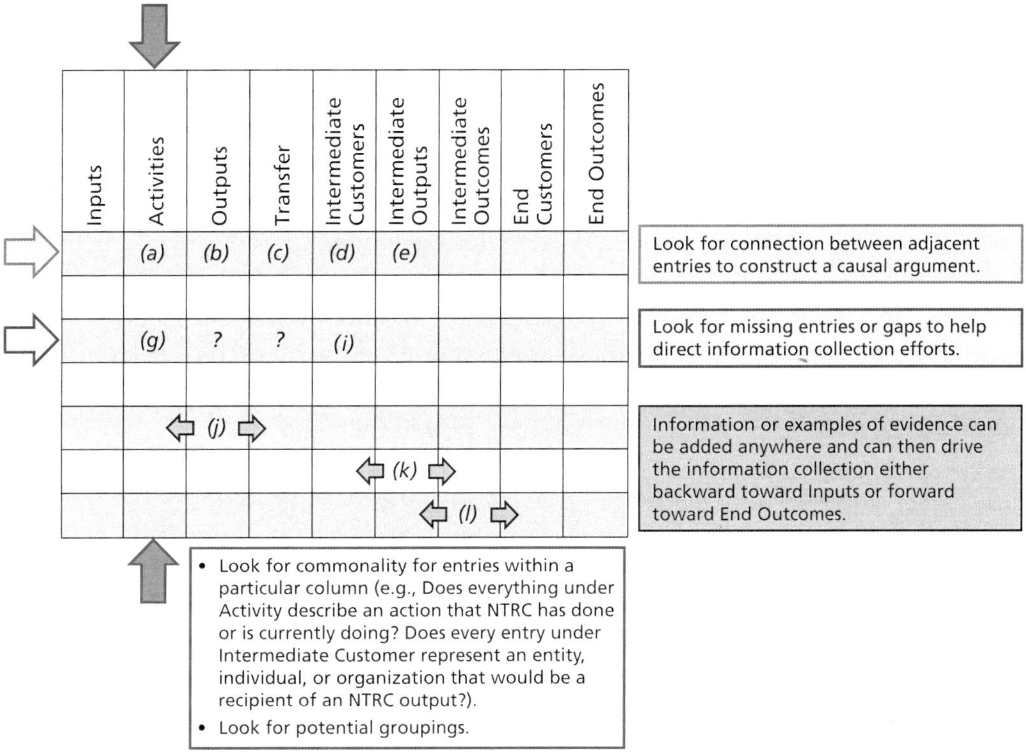

Inputs	Activities	Outputs	Transfer	Intermediate Customers	Intermediate Outputs	Intermediate Outcomes	End Customers	End Outcomes
	(a)	(b)	(c)	(d)	(e)			
	(g)	?	?	(i)				
	(j)							
				(k)				
					(l)			

Look for connection between adjacent entries to construct a causal argument.

Look for missing entries or gaps to help direct information collection efforts.

Information or examples of evidence can be added anywhere and can then drive the information collection either backward toward Inputs or forward toward End Outcomes.

- Look for commonality for entries within a particular column (e.g., Does everything under Activity describe an action that NTRC has done or is currently doing? Does every entry under Intermediate Customer represent an entity, individual, or organization that would be a recipient of an NTRC output?).
- Look for potential groupings.

SOURCE: Adapted from Williams et al. (2009).
RAND RR1108-A.3

classifications and to identify common themes among items for organizing or grouping information within a particular column.

One should also review the information across each row to identify and verify connections between adjacent cells. For example, did an activity yield an output that could be traced to a specific intermediate customer, and did that intermediate customer use that NTRC output to generate its own product or intermediate outputs? For example, is there a clear relationship between the contents of the cells labeled (a) through (e) in Figure A.3?

The process of horizontal inspection can also serve more than one purpose. It can provide a means to identify gaps, which, in turn, can drive a search for missing information. An NTRC activity that appears to jump to an intermediate customer without an obvious link (as illustrated in cells (g) and (i) in Figure A.3) raises the question: What output was generated, and how was it transferred or provided to the intermediate customer? This process can also be used to document the extent to which particular NTRC efforts have progressed to outcomes and to identify additional contacts in the search for evidence of impact. For instance, if a specific intermediate customer is known to have produced something from an NTRC output, it might be worth contacting that customer to learn if the customer has any evidence of how its products are being used (e.g., other companies or workers). Lastly, this process can also assist in constructing the many-to-many connection between activities and outputs to various outcomes. An NTRC activity or product can assist multiple intermediate and end customers and contribute to multiple intermediate outputs and outcomes. Moreover, multiple activities and outputs, over time, can cumulatively contribute to a single outcome that supports NIOSH's mission.

We provide a blank logic model worksheet template in Appendix C, along with a notional example of a partially completed logic model worksheet for one category of intermediate customers. In addition, individual elements from the present NTRC logic model, shown in Figure A.2, are presented in the next section. The current logic models, the various elements, and the specific entries within each element have been developed as part of the current pilot study, described in the main report. Each of these should be viewed as a starting point that can be appended (or modified) with additional entries or examples, pending future examinations of other portions of NTRC. It is reasonable to expect that additional inputs, activities, outputs, and intermediate customers—and even additional paths to outcomes—will be identified during reviews of additional portions of the center.

NTRC Inputs

In our approach to logic modeling, we typically categorize inputs as either production or planning inputs. Production inputs are the monetary, human, or physical resources needed for a program to function. Examples include dollars, people, and laboratory equipment. Planning inputs might include data or information that can mandate, direct, or lead to activities. Examples include legislation, strategic guidance, information about stakeholder needs or workplace risks (e.g., workplace surveillance data), information about new materials, and new information about known materials or risks (e.g., scientific articles). Table A.2 provides examples of the NTRC inputs that we identified during our document review.

NTRC Activities and Outputs

Table A.3 provides examples of NTRC activities and outputs. Activities represent what an organization does on a daily basis, and outputs are the direct, tangible products (e.g., guidance documents, prototypes) that the organization's activities generate.

Table A.2
Examples of NTRC Inputs

Inputs
Production
• Funding
• Staff
• Managerial support
• Laboratory and research facilities
Planning
• Budget, strategy, and planning documents
• Policies and plans
• Standards and guidance
• Needs or requests raised by stakeholders (e.g., partners, intermediate customers, and end customers)
• Risk assessment findings
• Scientific journal articles
• Animal and epidemiological studies

SOURCE: Based on RAND analysis of documents and stakeholder remarks, with input from NTRC.

NTRC Transfer

For many organizations, documenting evidence of contributions beyond outputs presents a significant challenge. For instance, it might be possible to monitor how often a particular presentation is made at scientific meetings or how many times a particular document is downloaded from the NIOSH website, but the exchange of information or knowledge that occurs through direct engagements with intermediate customers or workers is harder to track and quantify. Neither the time spent with intermediate customers nor the number of new findings shared with intermediate customers can fully reflect the potential value or contribution of this transfer mechanism for achieving outcomes. Nonetheless, the potential for this type of transfer to contribute to changes in workplace practices and enable intermediate and end outcomes is significant.[4] For this reason, the direct engagement of the field research teams is called out separately in the logic model shown in Figure A.2. Unlike other transfer mechanisms that we identified, direct engagement by the field research teams has the potential to impact final customers without having to pass through intermediate customers. Similarly, the direct engagement of NTRC staff and researchers with the center's diverse set of intermediate customers is an often-mentioned method for learning about NTRC activities and outputs, and therefore this method is highlighted first among the second set of transfer mechanisms (see Table A.4).

---

[4] The Howell, Silberglitt, and Norland (2003) report discusses the importance and value of on-site and direct engagement between the industry and researchers for finding effective solutions to industry-related problems. In addition, Section 2.6 of the *National Academies NIOSH Program Review: Health Hazard Evaluations* (CDC, 2007) discusses the transfer of information between NIOSH Health Hazard Evaluation response teams and staff working onsite at the workplace.

Table A.3
Examples of NTRC Activities and Outputs

Activities	Outputs
Conduct research	
• Research and evaluate the human health effects (e.g., pulmonary, respiratory, neuroimmune response, neurological) and toxicity associated with exposure to nanostructured materials (nanoparticles, nanotubes, nanofibers, and new forms of nanomaterials) • Research occupational exposures to nanostructured materials • Characterize the physical and chemical properties of nanostructured materials and products containing nanostructured materials • Characterize the transport mechanisms of nanostructured materials (e.g., aerosolized nanoparticles and nanowires) • Research and evaluate effectiveness of engineering controls and PPE for engineered nanomaterials	• Journal articles and scientific publications • Nanomaterials health and safety presentations
Develop instrumentation, test equipment, protocols, and reference materials	
• Develop equipment to generate and characterize dispersed or aerosolized nanoparticles • Identify and develop nanoscale reference materials for calibrating measurement instruments • Evaluate diffusion charge-based sensors • Develop protocol for measuring nanomaterial mass and surface area in animal inhalation chambers • Develop and evaluate nano-aerosol surface area measurement methods • Develop procedures to test and evaluate the effectiveness of PPE	• Design for aerosolized nanoparticle generator to test exposures • Technical input regarding nanostructured standard reference materials • Methods for measuring nanostructured materials' mass and surface area • NEAT • Draft standard for measuring mass and surface area of nanostructured materials
Conduct field assessments and monitor exposure	
• Conduct field research team site visits and exposure assessments • Assess occupational health risks associated with exposure to nanoscale materials • Analyze landscape of formulators and users of nanostructured materials • Contact and recruit companies for field assessments	• Site evaluation findings and reports • Survey of users and formulators of nanostructured materials • Method for health hazard banding for nanostructured materials where potential toxicity is unknown
Provide policy, guidance, and recommendations and facilitate coordination among customers and partners	
• Chair and participate on standards bodies and associations • Respond to comments on Current Intelligence Bulletins • Facilitate engagement among communities of interest	• Current Intelligence Bulletins • Recommended exposure limits • Recommended measurement methods • NIOSH numbered reports

SOURCE: Based on RAND analysis of documents and stakeholder remarks, with input from NTRC.

Table A.4
Examples of NTRC Transfer Mechanisms

Transfer
• Conduct field research team site visits with employers and employees at industries involved with the formulation or use of nanostructured materials
• Directly engage with customers • Publish scientific findings in journals • Publish and disseminate NIOSH numbered reports • Present at scientific and OSH conferences and meetings • Sponsor or co-sponsor workshops on engineered nanomaterials • Demonstrate equipment • Update the NIOSH blog

SOURCE: Based on RAND analysis of documents and stakeholder remarks, with input from NTRC.

NTRC Intermediate Customers and Intermediate Outputs

Examples of intermediate customers and corresponding intermediate outputs are shown in Table A.5. The types of intermediate outputs are not necessarily exclusive to a particular category. Both a research organization and an industry may publish updated procedures for handling nanomaterials. For clarity, it was instructive to align the categories of intermediate customer with the intermediate outputs that are representative of that category. This alignment process also highlights the multiple, different paths to achieving desired intermediate and end outcomes.

For intermediate customers, the industry category consists of manufacturers, distributors, fabricators and formulators, service industries, and manufacturers of instruments to monitor nanomaterials. Manufacturers are the companies that create or manufacture engineered nanomaterials. Distributors are companies that resell or distribute engineered nanomaterials to a broad range of customers. One way of thinking about the difference between formulators and fabricators is that a company that is a formulator is typically adding nanoparticles to a matrix where the nanoparticles will be held in suspension or distributed throughout the medium to provide enhanced or desirable properties, whereas fabricators integrate engineered nanomaterials as a discrete element or components of a device or structure. The fourth subcategory of industry includes service providers that use products that contain engineered nanomaterials. This subcategory also includes the growing number of companies involved with the recovery, recycling, or disposal of products that contain engineered nanomaterials. Manufacturers and designers of instruments to monitor and measure exposures to nanoscale materials can benefit from interactions with and outputs from NTRC when designing and developing these instruments for the workplace.

Advocacy refers broadly to groups or associations that might use NTRC outputs to create intermediate outputs to inform a target group or demographic, to advocate for a particular position, or to influence the views of policymakers, decisionmakers in industry, or others on a particular topic or issue.

Table A.5
Examples of NTRC Intermediate Customers and Corresponding Intermediate Outputs

Intermediate Customers	Intermediate Outputs
Industry (establish policies/procedures)	
• Manufacturers of nanomaterials • Distributors of nanomaterials • Fabricators and formulators that use nanomaterials • Service industries that use or encounter nanomaterials • Manufacturers of instruments to monitor and manipulate nanomaterials	• Modified engineering controls and PPE • Instrument for aerosol and hygiene sampling • Seminars and demos at site visits • Modified nano-enabled products • Revised safety data sheets • Patents • Papers
Advocacy	
• Business/industry associations • Law firms or legal organizations • Unions or worker representatives • Consensus standards groups • Other lobbyist groups • Other nongovernmental organizations	• Training materials • Trained workers • Training courses • Survey of workers • Responses to NIOSH RFIs • Conference presentations • Database of nano-enabled products • Standards committee studies • Information to raise awareness about OSH issues
Government (international, federal, state, local)	
• Regulators • Government laboratories and researchers • Technology transition offices	• CPSC risk assessment of products • EPA chemical notices • OSHA Fact Sheet • OSHA recommended exposure limits • NIST protocols on nanomaterial preparation • Publications and research findings • Patents • Updates to 40 C.F.R. Part 721 • Research strategy documents • NIST Standard Reference Materials
Researchers and research institutions	
• Individual researchers • Academic research institutions • Other nongovernmental laboratories	• Publications and research findings • Updated nanomaterial handling procedures • Enhanced awareness of exposure assessments • Enhanced credibility with industry • Patents
Education and training	
• Universities • Training institutions • Trainers	• Training materials • Trained workers

SOURCE: Intermediate customers were based on NIOSH documents and Sayes (2013, 2014), with input from NTRC. Intermediate outputs were based on analysis of other documents and stakeholder remarks, with input from NTRC.

Government intermediate customers are the various federal, state, and local government agencies and offices that use NTRC's outputs. At the federal level, these include, for example, other government laboratories, such as NIST; government regulatory and research organizations, such as EPA and OSHA; and other offices and programs within and across NIOSH.

Researchers and research institutions are the individual researchers, universities, nongovernmental laboratories, think-tanks, and so on that might use NTRC research findings, scientific articles, or publications (outputs) to inform their current research and to shape their research agendas. Moreover, they might refer to the NTRC outputs in their own academic articles or publications.

Intermediate customers involved with developing or providing education and training might also be involved in research, but, in this capacity, they might use NTRC outputs to produce training materials, create new engineering practices or procedures, and train individuals. Individuals could, for example, be trained in occupational or environmental health and safety practices and procedures related, in part or whole, directly or indirectly, to nanomaterials. OSHA, some universities, and other organizations, such as organized labor, have or are affiliated with training or certification programs in occupational and environmental health and safety that might pertain to nanomaterials. However, according to NTRC staff, education and training in the handling and potential risks of engineered nanomaterials in the workplace also occur in laboratories that are training researchers and staff who are exposed to engineered nanomaterials through their work. As the number and variety of companies working with engineered nanomaterials expands, those NTRC customers who engage with education and training might be of increasing importance in helping NTRC connect with industry to increase the number of trained specialists who are implementing enhanced practices and procedures for the safe handling of engineered nanomaterials.

NTRC Intermediate Outcomes, End Customers, and End Outcomes

Table A.6 lists examples of both the NTRC intermediate outcomes that are connected to or derived from the intermediate outputs presented in Table A.5 and the notional paths for achieving desired outcomes.

Typically, as one gets further away from an organization's activities and outputs (program efforts) and closer to the organization's end customers and end outcomes (program effects), it becomes more difficult to distinguish how the organization's efforts have contributed to change as separate from the contributions of other organizations and actors. For research organizations like NIOSH that rely heavily on intermediate customers to achieve their missions, it can be especially difficult to document specific evidence that suggests impact. This can be true for several reasons, including the fact that it can take many years for research outputs to move along the path to end outcomes. It might also be the case that the surveillance or monitoring necessary to

Table A.6
Examples of NTRC End Customers and Notional Intermediate and End Outcomes

Intermediate Outcomes	End Customers	Intermediate Outcomes	End Outcomes
• Acquisition of engineering controls and PPE in industrial processes • Acquisition and use of nano-enabled construction materials • Use of NIOSH-developed measure methods • Use of NIST Standard Reference Materials • Acquisition of monitoring and sampling equipment	• Workers • Supervisors • Managers and business owners	• Adoption and use of PPE, engineering controls, and changes in processes • Reduced exposure to engineered nanomaterials	• Reduction in work-related illness and injuries related to engineered nanomaterials

SOURCE: Based on RAND analysis, with input from NTRC.

document or measure changes along the path is missing or unobtainable; absent that capability, it might be difficult, if not impossible, to isolate a contribution.

For added emphasis, we restate that NTRC field research teams provide an alternative means of directly transferring NTRC outputs to end customers, without needing intermediate customers and intermediate outcomes. Also, in this case, we note that end customer "workers" are not limited to employees in the industry; this category may also refer to researchers at academic or government laboratories who are handling and working with engineered nanomaterials.

Identify and Contact NTRC Stakeholders

Using the foundation created in the previous section, Step 4 in the process is to select stakeholders (including intermediate customers, end customers, and partners) to contact to validate the perceived model of how NTRC is contributing to outcomes, to collect additional examples of intermediate outputs and outcomes, and to document alternative paths to achieving outcomes.

We suggest the following criteria for identifying potential stakeholders to contact:

- Potential contacts should fall within the scope the assessment.
- They, or the organizations they represent, should be mentioned or referenced in the documents that have been collected or be identified by another intermediate customer.
- Taken in combination, they should collectively span the relevant categories of intermediate customers, end customers, and partners.

Each type of customer will use NTRC outputs in a different way and to produce different types of intermediate outputs, as described in Table A.5. In addition, partners may engage with NTRC in ways different from customers. Therefore, we suggest identifying a diverse set of intermediate customers and stakeholders to learn about how they use NTRC outputs to contribute to outcomes.

For each proposed contact, we recommend completing a logic model worksheet with the information at hand, to briefly summarize how NTRC's program efforts (e.g., inputs, activities, outputs, and transfers) are used by that particular intermediate customer to produce program effects. This step is useful for familiarizing oneself with the products of the intermediate customer and its relationship with NTRC, and the worksheet can help guide discussions. Notional logic model worksheets are provided in Appendix C.

We recommend holding conversations in person or by phone. Because of differences in how contacts might define or think about certain terms (such as *impact*), we suggest direct engagement, or direct engagement in concert with other broader survey methods, for this type of exercise. Through direct contact, it is more possible to get all participants on the same page, using terms consistently.

The length of each conversation and the level of detail can be expected to vary, but common themes should include the customer's general familiarity with NIOSH and NTRC; familiarity with NTRC outputs (e.g., research findings, recommendations, other publications, services); how the customer becomes aware of or obtains NTRC outputs; how they use those outputs, including how they share them with other customers, peers, and partners; and how NTRC outputs affect their own products, services, or practices. It might also be worth inquiring whether the contact would recommend reaching out to any other individuals or organizations.

Example of the types of information that might be collected include the implementation of changes to workplace practices or procedures, the development of information or policy statements, changes in research topics, inclusion of NTRC findings in ongoing research efforts, and the development of new training materials or curricula.

The purpose of the conversations is, *ultimately*, to uncover information about how NTRC program efforts are contributing to desired outcomes.

Refine NTRC Logic Model and Develop Outcome Narratives

The final step in our logic modeling process involves reviewing the findings from the previous step and then revising the NTRC logic model, as needed, to fill in any gaps. There are several valid approaches to completing this last step. One recommendation is to review the notes from each discussion and highlight examples of transfer, intermediate outputs, and contributions to outcomes that were mentioned during the discussion. It can also be helpful to capture any other issues, observations, or external factors that contacts suggest might be enhancing or inhibiting NTRC's contributions to outcomes. A useful (but not required) next step would be to update the individual intermediate customer logic model worksheets for future reference. These documents might also be used to develop narratives of how NTRC is contributing to outcomes.[5] To complete the process, we recommend updating the NTRC logic model to reflect the findings.

The entire process can be repeated for other portions of NTRC, for other NIOSH components, or for the same portion over time.

---

[5] A comprehensive description of the process of converting logic model worksheets to outcome narratives is available in Williams et al. (2009), Chapter Five.

NIOSH Logic Model

Figure B.1
NIOSH Logic Model and Mission

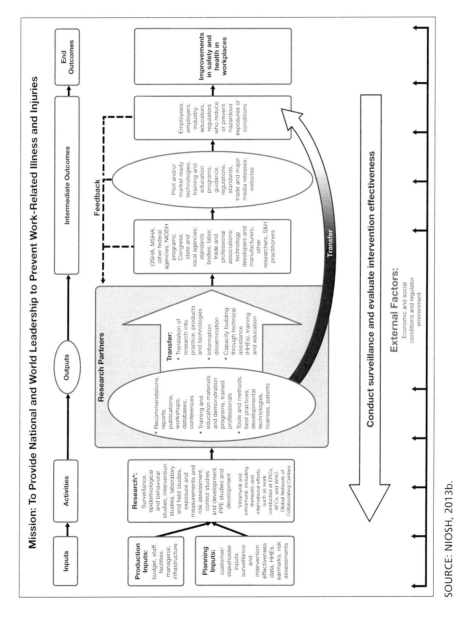

SOURCE: NIOSH, 2013b.
NOTE: HHE = Health Hazard Evaluation; ERC = Education and Research Center; WHO = World Health Organization;
MSHA = Mine Safety and Health Administration; S&H = shipping and handling.
RAND RR1108-B.1

Notional Logic Model Worksheets

This appendix includes an example of a blank logic model worksheet that can be used for recording and organizing information about inputs through outcomes (Table C.1).

It also includes a notional example of a partially completed worksheet (Table C.2). The information shown is notional and for illustrative purposes. However, the examples in the individual cells are informed by NIOSH's documentation and discussions with various NTRC customers.

Table C.1
Blank Logic Model Worksheet

Source or Reference	Inputs	Activities	Outputs	Transfers	Intermediate Customers	Intermediate Outputs	Intermediate Outcomes	End Customers	(Intermediate Outcomes)	End Outcomes

SOURCE: Adapted from Greenfield, Williams, and Eiseman (2006) and Williams et al. (2009).

Table C.2
Sample Notional Logic Model Worksheet: Industry

Source or Reference	Inputs	Activities	Outputs	Transfers	Intermediate Customers	Intermediate Outputs	Intermediate Outcomes	End Customers	(Intermediate Outcomes)	End Outcomes
NIOSH numbered document	Equipment to measure nanoparticles in air samples	Evaluate nanoparticle sampling equipment and algorithms	Techniques and methods for monitoring nanoparticle exposure	NTRC field research teams use equipment and methods to evaluate occupational settings	N/A[a]	N/A[a]	N/A[a]	Managers; Workers in occupational settings	Changes in workplace practices	
		Research respirator test-fit using nanoparticle sampling equipment	Scientific publications	Briefings at scientific meetings; Publications in scientific OSH-related journals						
NIOSH document	Identified gaps in nanomaterial toxicity	Research toxicity for specific nanomaterial	Research findings and recommended exposure limit for specific nanomaterial	Direct engagement with industry; Published to NIOSH website	Nanomaterial manufacturer	Updated employer nanomaterial handling practices	N/A	Managers; Workers in occupational settings	Changes in workplace practices	

SOURCE: Adapted by RAND staff.

[a] N/A = not applicable; in this case, the transfer occurs directly to end customers.

Bibliography

Bartis, James T., and Eric Landree, *Nanomaterials in the Workplace: Policy and Planning Workshop on Occupational Safety and Health*, Santa Monica, Calif.: RAND Corporation, CF-227-NIOSH, 2006. As of December 12, 2014:
http://www.rand.org/pubs/conf_proceedings/CF227.html

CDC—*See* Centers for Disease Control and Prevention.

Centers for Disease Control and Prevention, *National Academies NIOSH Program Review: Health Hazard Evaluations*, 2007. As of December 14, 2014:
http://www.cdc.gov/niosh/nas/hhe/

———, *About NIOSH*, 2013a. As of December 14, 2014:
http://www.cdc.gov/niosh/about.html

———, *National Academies Evaluation of NIOSH Programs*, 2013b. As of May 15, 2015:
http://www.cdc.gov/niosh/nas/

———, *NIOSH Program Portfolio*, 2013c. As of May 12, 2015:
http://www.cdc.gov/niosh/programs/default.html

———, *NIOSH Regulations*, 2013d. As of May 12, 2015:
http://www.cdc.gov/niosh/regulations.html

———, *Nanotechnology: Overview*, October 6, 2014. As of February 23, 2015:
http://www.cdc.gov/niosh/topics/nanotech/

———, *Directory of NIOSH Offices and Key Personnel*, 2015a. As of May 12, 2015:
http://www.cdc.gov/niosh/contact/officers.html

———, *Funding*, 2015b. As of October 7, 2015:
http://www.cdc.gov/funding/

Greenfield, Victoria A., Valerie L. Williams, and Elisa Eiseman, *Using Logic Models for Strategic Planning and Evaluation: Application to the National Center for Injury Prevention and Control*, Santa Monica, Calif.: RAND Corporation, TR-370-NCIPC, 2006. As of December 14, 2014:
http://www.rand.org/pubs/technical_reports/TR370.html

Greenfield, Victoria A., Henry H. Willis, and Tom LaTourrette, *Assessing the Benefits of U.S. Customs and Border Protection Regulatory Actions to Reduce Terrorism Risks*, Santa Monica, Calif.: RAND Corporation, CF-301-INDEC, 2012. As of December 14, 2014:
http://www.rand.org/pubs/conf_proceedings/CF301.html

Howell, David R., Richard Silberglitt, and Douglas Norland, *Industrial Materials for the Future R&D Strategies: A Case Study of Boiler Materials for the Pulp and Paper Industry*, Santa Monica, Calif.: RAND Corporation, MR-1583-NREL, 2003. As of December 14, 2014:
http://www.rand.org/pubs/monograph_reports/MR1583.html

McLaughlin, J. G., and G. B. Jordan, "Logic Models: A Tool for Telling Your Program's Performance Story," *Evaluation and Program Planning*, Vol. 22, No. 1, 1999, pp. 65–72.

Mitton, C., C. E. Adair, E. McKenzie, S. B. Patten, and B. W. Perry, "Knowledge Transfer and Exchange: Review and Synthesis of the Literature," *Milbank Quarterly*, Vol. 85, No. 4, 2007, pp. 729–768.

National Institute for Occupational Safety and Health, *Current Intelligence Bulletin 60: Interim Guidance for Medical Screening and Hazard Surveillance for Workers Potentially Exposed to Engineered Nanomaterials,* Cincinnati, Ohio: U.S. Department of Health and Human Services, Centers for Disease Control and Prevention, National Institute for Occupational Safety and Health, DHHS (NIOSH) Publication No. 2009-116, February 2009a. As of December 12, 2014:
http://www.cdc.gov/niosh/docs/2009-116/

———, *Approaches to Safe Nanotechnology: Managing the Health and Safety Concerns Associated with Engineered Nanomaterials*, Cincinnati, Ohio: U.S. Department of Health and Human Services, Centers for Disease Control and Prevention, National Institute for Occupational Safety and Health, DHHS (NIOSH) Publication No. 2009-125, March 2009b. As of December 12, 2014:
http://www.cdc.gov/niosh/docs/2009-125/

———, *Current Intelligence Bulletin 63: Occupational Exposure to Titanium Dioxide.* Cincinnati, Ohio: U.S. Department of Health and Human Services, Centers for Disease Control and Prevention, National Institute for Occupational Safety and Health, DHHS (NIOSH) Publication No. 2011-160, 2011. As of December 12, 2014:
http://www.cdc.gov/niosh/docs/2011-160/

———, *Filling the Knowledge Gap for Safe Nanotechnology in the Workplace, A Progress Report from the NIOSH Nanotechnology Research Center, 2004–2011.* Cincinnati, Ohio: U.S. Department of Health and Human Services, Centers for Disease Control and Prevention, National Institute for Occupational Safety and Health, DHHS (NIOSH) Publication No. 2013-101, 2012a. As of August 30, 2015:
http://www.cdc.gov/niosh/docs/2013-101/pdfs/2013-101.pdf

———, *General Safe Practices for Working with Engineered Nanomaterials in Research Laboratories*, Cincinnati, Ohio: U.S. Department of Health and Human Services, Centers for Disease Control and Prevention, National Institute for Occupational Safety and Health, DHHS (NIOSH) Publication No. 2012-147, 2012b. As of December 12, 2014:
http://www.cdc.gov/niosh/docs/2012-147/

———, *Current Intelligence Bulletin 65: Occupational Exposure to Carbon Nanotubes and Nanofibers*, Cincinnati, Ohio: U.S. Department of Health and Human Services, Centers for Disease Control and Prevention, National Institute for Occupational Safety and Health, DHHS (NIOSH) Publication No. 2013-145, 2013a. As of December 12, 2014:
http://www.cdc.gov/niosh/docs/2013-145/

———, *Protecting the Nanotechnology Workforce: NIOSH Nanotechnology Research and Guidance Strategic Plan, 2013–2016*, Cincinnati, Ohio: U.S. Department of Health and Human Services, Centers for Disease Control and Prevention, National Institute for Occupational Safety and Health, DHHS (NIOSH) Publication 2014-106, 2013b. As of December 12, 2014:
http://www.cdc.gov/niosh/docs/2014-106/

National Science and Technology Council, *National Nanotechnology Initiative: Supplement to the President's 2016 Budget*, Washington, D.C.: National Science and Technology Council, Committee on Technology, Subcommittee on Nanoscale Science, Engineering, and Technology, March 2015. As of May 13, 2015:
http://www.nano.gov/sites/default/files/pub_resource/nni_fy16_budget_supplement.pdf

NIOSH—*See* National Institute for Occupational Safety and Health.

Occupational Safety and Health Administration, "Working Safely with Nanomaterials," *OSHA Fact Sheet*, U.S. Department of Labor, DTSEM FS-3634, 2013. As of August 30, 2015:
https://www.osha.gov/Publications/OSHA_FS-3634.pdf

Public Law 91-173, Federal Mine Safety and Health Act of 1977, as amended by Public Law 95-164, November 9, 1977.

Public Law 91-596, Occupational Safety and Health Act of 1970, December 29, 1970.

Public Law 113-235, Division G, Title II—Department of Health and Human Services. National Institute for Occupational Safety and Health, December 16, 2014.

Rauwel, Protima, Erwan Rauwel, Stanislav Ferdov, and Mangala P. Singh, "Silver Nanoparticles: Synthesis, Properties, and Applications," *Advances in Materials Science and Engineering*, Vol. 2015, 2015.

Ruegg, Rosalie, and Gretchen Jordan, *Overview of Evaluation Methods for R&D Programs: A Directory of Evaluation Methods Relevant to Technology Development Programs*, Prepared for the U.S. Department of Energy, Office of Energy Efficiency and Renewable Energy, 2007. As of May 18, 2015:
https://www1.eere.energy.gov/analysis/pdfs/evaluation_methods_r_and_d.pdf

Sayes, Christie, *NanoSurveillance: Commonly Used Engineered Nanomaterials in the United States: A Market Landscape Analysis*, Research Triangle Park, N.C.: RTI International, RTI Project Number 0212288.013, 2013.

———, *Conduct a Secondary Value Market Landscape Survey on Nanoscale Cellulose, Silver, Titanium Dioxide, and Graphene: A Market Landscape Analysis*, Research Triangle Park, N.C.: RTI International, RTI Project Number 0212288.017, 2014.

Shadish, William R., Thomas D. Cook, Laura C. Leviton, *Foundations of Program Evaluation: Theories of Practice*, Newbury Park, Calif.: Sage Publications, Inc., 1991.

Taylor-Powell, Ellen, and Ellen Henert, *Developing a Logic Model: Teaching and Training Guide*, Madison, Wisc.: University of Wisconsin–Extension, Cooperative Extension, 2008. As of December 14, 2014:
http://www.uwex.edu/ces/pdande/evaluation/pdf/lmguidecomplete.pdf

Wholey, Joseph S., Harry P. Hatry, and Kathryn E. Newcomer, eds., *Handbook of Practical Program Evaluation*, 3rd ed., San Francisco, Calif.: Jossey-Bass and Imprint of Wiley, 2010.

Williams, Valerie L., Elisa Eiseman, Eric Landree, and David M. Adamson, *Demonstrating and Communicating Research Impact: Preparing NIOSH Programs for External Review*, Santa Monica, Calif.: RAND Corporation, MG-809-NIOSH, 2009. As of December 12, 2014:
http://www.rand.org/pubs/monographs/MG809.html

W.K. Kellogg Foundation, *Logic Model Development Guide*, Battle Creek, Mich., 2006. As of December 14, 2014:
http://www.wkkf.org/resource-directory/resource/2006/02/
wk-kellogg-foundation-logic-model-development-guide